Letters to Myself
Volume 6
Emotional, Physical, & Spiritual Wellbeing

By:
Award Winning
&
#1 International Bestselling Author
Jen Taylor, LCSW

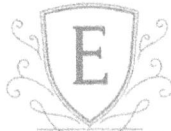

E

ELITE PUBLISHING
HOUSE
YOUR LEGACY. YOUR BOOK.

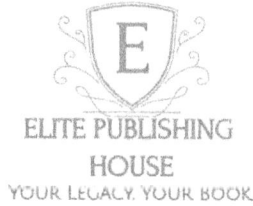

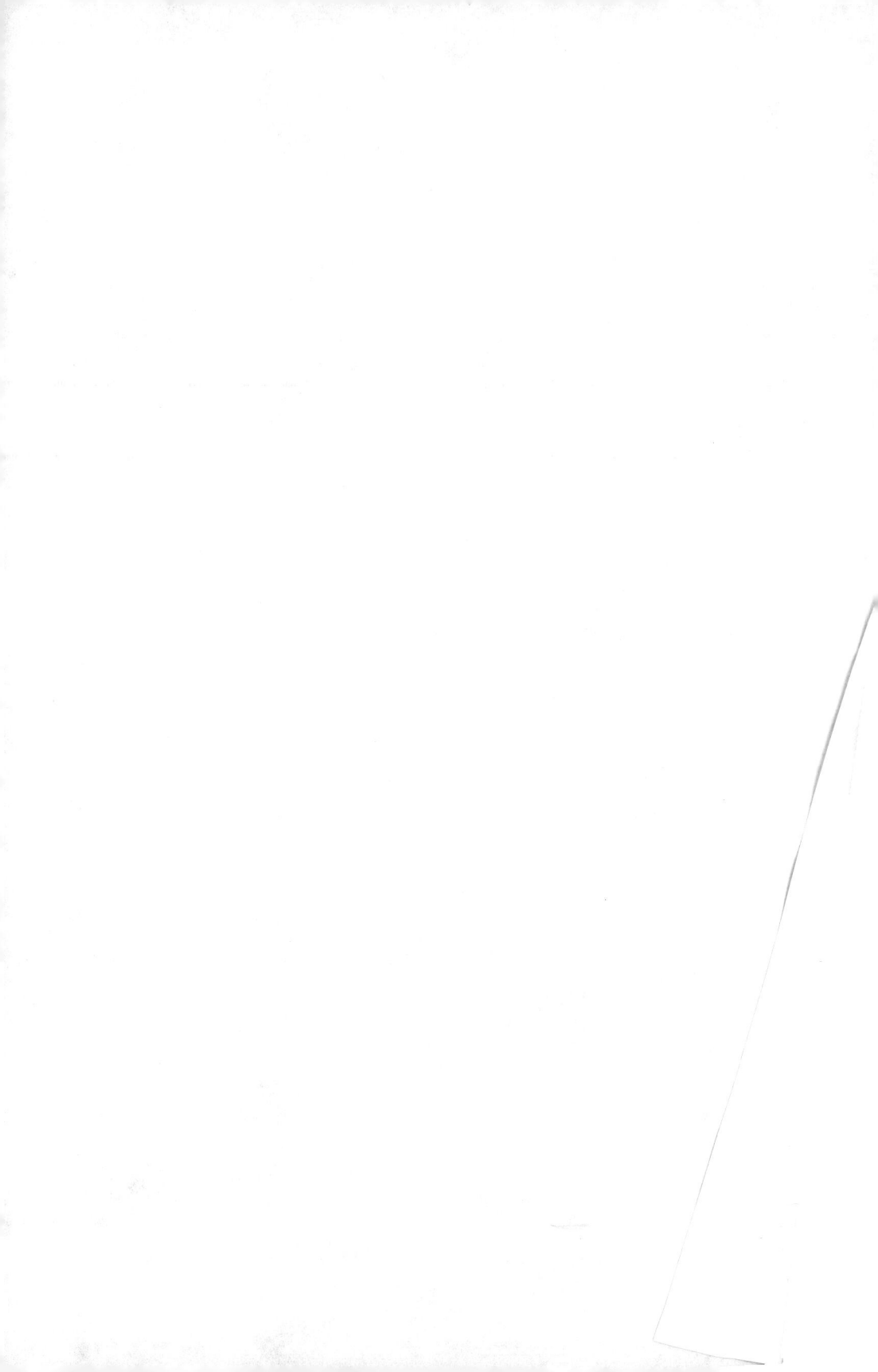

To my kids, Giancarlo & Elisabetta, my "pezzi di core."

Thank you both for all you have taught me and

for choosing me to be your mom.

United States:

If you or someone you know is experiencing a mental health, suicide crisis, or emotional distress, reach out 24/7 to the 988 Suicide and Crisis Lifeline (formerly known as the National Suicide Prevention Lifeline) by dialing or texting 988 or using chat services at suicidepreventionlifeline.org to connect to a trained crisis counselor.

Please see Appendix Suicide Resources for Worldwide Numbers

Mental Health:

NAMI Helpline (National Alliance on Mental Illness) 1-800-950-6264

TABLE OF CONTENTS

FOREWORD

Demitra Vassiliadis

Spiritual/Astrologer

When Jen asked me to write the intro for this volume on emotional, physical, and spiritual well-being, I was both honored and daunted. I am not a doctor, naturopath, healer, or psychologist, so I cannot offer professional insights on these fronts. I have been on my own healing journey for most of my life, and the issue of our collective well-being is often at the forefront of my mind, as is the epidemic of mental, physical, and spiritual sickness that plagues us in the modern world.

It is my observation that most, if not all, illness stems from a rupture in our relationship to Source, our parents, or our families, to the authentic self, to each other, or to the natural world and creation. Therefore, any true healing must address how to reconnect in a meaningful way. To heal implies to be made whole. To be made whole implies something, somewhere, broke or was ruptured.

As a Spiritual Astrologer, I view life through the prism of Spiritual Astrology, which posits that we are all sacred beings created by the same majestic, infinite love that authored the stars, planets, and all of creation. Our ultimate well-being flows from that Source, and when ruptured, can be re-established by remembering our sacred origin and reconnecting with Spirit. Astrology can help heal our spiritual amnesia by reminding us that our presence here on earth is not random but aligned with the perfect astrological moment for our evolution and to make our unique contribution while we are here incarnated. This perspective goes far in healing the profound alienation that is the cause of so much sickness.

This remembering restores not only our right relationship to the Source and the cosmos but also our sense of soul purpose, which steers us back to sanity and sacredness. While our physical health and well-being can feel most primary in the triad of mind, body, and Spirit, it is the spiritual connection that is, in fact, the most primal. When our spirits leave our bodies, we die to this life.

Volumes could be written on spiritual practices and techniques, and there are no doubt as many practices as there are people. It is not my intention to instruct the readers of this introduction on the particulars of spiritual practice but to merely recommend finding one that works to establish inner peace and a connection to Source. My own practice includes daily prayer, meditation, and time outdoors. I have found that when I put my spiritual well-being first, everything else falls more or less into place, or I can find peace or acceptance with painful, trying circumstances.

Astrologically, our emotional well-being is tied primarily to the Moon, the maternal luminary of feelings, and the needs they point to. This indicates that our primary sense of emotional well-being is informed by our experience in the womb and how we bond with our mother or primary caregiver in infancy. Volumes could be written about the many societal, medical, and traumatic occurrences that have altered or ruptured the organic relationship and natural bonding of mother and child in the modern world, to say nothing of the emotional disruption caused by social media that has replaced traditional human bonding. Additionally, our minds are increasingly influenced by social media, which captures our attention and points us outward to seek approval and connection on the internet rather than seeking connection within and with human connection to friends, family, and nature.

We are challenged to learn to repair ruptured or traumatic attachment patterns and heal emotional traumas, which can be done through support groups, inner child work, somatic work, and through new emerging technologies in the Aquarian Age like EMDR (Eye Movement desensitization reprogramming), Emotional Freedom Technique Internal Family System, and learning simple methods of self-soothing and a daily self-care practice.

The body is the final frontier in the well-being triad, a living temple that records and responds to our experiences. From the Spiritual Astrology perspective, the Universe incarnates through each of us. As the great Sufi poet Rumi wrote: You are not a drop in the ocean; you are the entire sea in a drop. This sacred perspective on the body can help us overcome the relentless objectification and degrading exploitation that pop culture inflicts on the human body and our perception of it.

The human body is currently assaulted with chemicals, drugs, alcohol, processed food, and an epidemic of PTSD.

Spiritual Astrology reminds us that the body is a microcosm of the heavens that houses our souls and the planetary forces. Each of our 7 chakras is a center for one of the visible to the eye 7 planets that connect us to limitless energy. This energy, properly understood and mastered through practices like yoga, Tai Chi,

Chi gong, or meditation, can lead us to higher states of consciousness and enlightenment.

Reclaiming the body through self-acceptance, somatic healing modalities, and a deeper understanding of the sacred and universal dimension that the body houses can go a long way to healing our embodied experience. A simple daily practice of blessing our bodies can work wonders and shift us out of negativity and criticism of our bodies.

Perhaps the most healing effect Astrology has had on me is that it restores a sense of meaning to life. We are all on the Hero/Heroines journey from the Astrological perspective. We all have dragons to face and our inner gold, symbolic of our unique talents and the authentic self, to be discovered and recovered. At this time, for many, certainly, for those contributing to this volume, the Healing Journey is the Hero's/heroine's journey, a noble pursuit well worth taking. Astrology provides a mythic meaning that can make sense of and enable acceptance of the suffering required on the healing journey. We are reminded that as we heal ourselves, we heal our world and light the way for those who follow.

In Solidarity with those on the Healing Journey,

-Demitra Vassiliadis
Spiritual/Astrologer
Contact Info:
heaventoearthastrology.com
heaventoearthastrology@gmail.com

INTRODUCTION

Emotional, physical & spiritual well-being

When I thought of wellness or well-being as a kid, I mostly thought of physical health. That was way back in the 1970s. Emotional well-being appeared in my 20s when I began therapy. The concept of spiritual WB arose during my college studies of Nagarjuna Buddhism with Ashok Gangadean, PhD. and again, at around age 32 - when I was pregnant with my first child. I was always a spiritual being - from a young age - I just didn't know what that meant or what to do with it. The concept that these are all interrelated made sense, but it wasn't until recently that emotional WB was considered - particularly in the workplace. It was as if, upon entering work, we had to "hang up" our emotional and spiritual parts and just do the job.

Two of the most outstanding individuals and supervisors in my social work/therapy world blessed me with incorporating these three parts. Firstly, Lauren Lesser, LCSW-R, Psy…who always checked in on a human level before discussing clients and cases. I vividly remember one thing that she said to me during my first year as a working therapist: "You never know how what you say will impact a client. It might be years later when they recall something you said that comforted them or provided hope." and "for some of these kids, you being a consistent and loving adult who listens to them is the greatest gift." My second blessing of a supervisor, Rosalie Wilson, LCSW-R, always checked in with me first, "Jen - on a scale of 1-10, how are you doing?" as well as her famous saying that I reference to this day, "No plan is a plan without a backup." Both of these wise women understood that I was a therapist *and* a mom. Sometimes, Jen, the therapist, had to take the back burner to Jen, the mom.

We are souls living on the physical plane, and with our bodies come complications of physical disease and wellness. Our minds may be burdened with disease as well, including but not limited to anxiety, depression, etc. Our minds have an intense power to create well-being, as CBT (cognitive behavioral therapy) reminds us - that thoughts create feelings.

I have had the honor of working with spiritual teachers since my 20s, and to this day, my teacher and friend, Elizabeth Myers, reflects my gifts back to me and helps guide me on the way of my soul. My good friends are intuitive healers, astrologers, therapists, and doulas of both life and death. I never doubted the existence of the soul, and its undeniable presence was confirmed to me when my mother passed over. On Mother's Day of 2015, my brother and I felt the palpable absence of my mother's soul - a profound emptiness that echoed throughout her home.

Our authors, both anonymous and named, have courageously shared their letters and stories of their lives - physical ailments, emotional challenges, and spiritual awakenings. I am indebted to them for birthing this volume, for breathing life into an idea, a wish, a dream.

If you struggle with chronic illness, many of which are unseen, like CRPS, fibromyalgia, chronic pain, MS, crippling anxiety, OCD, depression, bipolar disorder, suicidal or intrusive thoughts, crises of faith, dark nights of the soul...please read on. Allow us to take you on a journey of overcoming, seeing the "light at the end of the tunnel," and restoring hope that may have been lost along the way.

Thank you to my dear Demitra Vassiliadis, spiritual astrologer, for offering to share her wisdom and eloquence of spoken and written word in the introduction. Amelia Denhof has brought this series alive with her stunning graphics. Lastly, Blair Hayse of Elite Publishing House has always had words of encouragement when I doubted if this would ever happen.

Thank you, dear reader, for taking the time (our most precious commodity) to read Volume 6.

-Jen Taylor, LCSW

COLLECTION OF LETTERS

"See, fatso is here; she has gained more weight as if she is planning for sumo wrestling."

"How ugly she looks, dark fat one."

"Uhh, a swollen egg, naah, let me correct a rotten egg."

"Good that she is alone; otherwise, she would have embarrassed her partner."

In social settings, these were the comments I usually heard for myself. 2018, it was a second year of suffering from Pemphigus. I was diagnosed with this skin autoimmune in August 2017. Since then, they kept me on steroids. It took six months to recover from blisters and skin burns. Unfortunately, autoimmune never had a concrete treatment in allopathic treatment or in alternative medicine practices. Steroids are the only help, but they are not toll-free. They destroy something while curing the autoimmune. Heavy loss of calcium, excessive weight gain, hair fall, numb muscle numbness, delayed menstrual cycle, less bleeding time, and memory loss are all a la carte things.

Medico advised me to stay forever on steroids with reduced strength once the skin gets cured. As days passed, my skin was getting cured, and other things started affecting me. My size changed from Xl to 4Xl. Those days, seeing myself in the mirror was the most disheartening thing. Not only was I losing physical strength, but I was losing my mental strength, too. My bedroom was the only square where nobody was allowed to enter and see my suffering. Quick cooking or bathing time was the only time I visited other places in the house. Those were the days of social disconnect. I never wanted to gather fake sympathies and uninvited advice from anyone.

Aloofness was killing me. Some days went all okay, and a few others were nightmares. After these six months of a rollercoaster ride, the remission period started. But I had lost the zeal to be social again. Most of us perceive ourselves in the eyes of society. If they praise us, we will maintain confidence. Otherwise, we self-doubt our abilities. I was doing exactly the same. I found escaping was the easiest way. It was the one way I knew I would neither face someone or someone would question me.

Depression and anxiety attacks started encountering me at less frequent intervals. A lively girl is now an old-looking lady. At the age of thirty-three, I started looking like I was fifty. Life's plan served me with this undesirable transformation.

I have always been a fighter by spirit, but I lost it. My fighter spirit was feeble but meekly poking my consciousness that this is not the way I am. Circumstances can be the wrath of destiny, but this is not long-lasting.

"Can I have a word with you?" my father asked.

"Ya sure, Papa," I nodded.

"Don't do this to yourself. This can't be you. Losing a game or a battle is okay, but labeling yourself a loser is not right. My daughter is a fighter."

I smiled for the first time in months. His advice restored my faith.

I started going out for a short period. Stepping out into public or social settings was not as easy as it looked. I had to face

18

insensitive voices who mocked my presence near me. These vilifying comments aggravated the pain inside me.

The remission period of autoimmune lasted for a couple of months, with steroid treatment going simultaneously. Life was not normal. Memory jerks were there. Overheating or burning of food in the kitchen was an every second-day story. A couple of times, I forgot the reason for what I was doing at a particular place during my outing. It took me a few minutes to recall. Steroids were making me clumsier day by day.

It was a strong tussle between physical and mental wrath, which I was losing. I never found it a great idea to share my medical condition with my social circle. Maybe I am a sympathetic person or want to talk less about the topic. I believe it's better to be together than to show fake sympathy and never look back.

Society always had an issue with being empathic toward people. On one such fateful day, when I was out to the temple for prayers, I met an acquaintance there. "Oh, you were left alone in life with these ugly scars. Your boyfriend must have left you due to it," she said in front of everyone in the temple. This nasty comment created a buzz, and everyone started looking at me with weird expressions. Tears began falling in a second. I was emotionally vulnerable, and this socially embarrassing moment engulfed my sanity once again. My failed relationship and disease can be a subject of mockery, or my life's struggle can be gossip, for gossip mongers set me in the deepest sorrows. Within the next few days, the autoimmune started relapsing once again. This time, it ruptured like a pandemic in no time. Things started to worsen and worsen in every passing moment. This time, the doctor suggested immediate admission to the hospital and heavy steroid infusions. This was a re-start to a painful experience once again.

I was back to square one with high intensity. The burning sensation on my skin, the pain, and hiding myself in the room were some setbacks. One day, when I pulled off my t-shirt, my skin pulled off because of sticky pus, and blood started oozing out. My father heard me whining and entered the room. It was the first time he saw my bare back with skin ruptures. He applied medicine all over with tears in his eyes. I was feeling ashamed that I had to face my father in such a helpless situation. It's highly unsettling to see a parent cry. The man who always provided me with a secure environment was getting weak. For a moment, I felt it was more painful than my autoimmune disorder. That was a moment of realization for me. I knew I had to get up for my old, powerful man. I didn't have any other option for myself.

I started playing meditative music on my mobile and chanting mantras. Divine interventions were required to regain mental strength. Within a month, I started feeling a little better, but still, I mostly lay on my bed. This time, instead of whining, I was listening to lectures. My second year Master's exam was pending. I couldn't think of writing a paper in such dizziness and pain. Still, I almost completed my course with freely available podcasts and videos available at public libraries on the internet. It was 31st December, and the year would change in mere moments. People were merrily spending the last moments of the year. I woke at 8AM, changed my clothes, and covered myself properly. It took me one hour to do so. While preparing the tea vessels in the kitchen, my father woke up. On routine winter days, he usually got up late. He asked me, "Are you okay, going to see the doctor?"

20

"No, Papa, I have an exam today."

"Leave it and take care of your health first," he commanded

"Let me try at least. I want to do it."

"How will you go? Do you have any preparations?"

"I took online classes. Even if I fail; I want to write it today."

"Then give me a few minutes. I will accompany you to the exam center."

"No, Papa, I will go. After all, I am your fighter girl."

"Oh, shut up, and stop being kiddish."

"You stop being so judgmental. You always taught me to face every toughness with grace. Then why are you stopping me today?"

He remained silent.

I poured tea into cups and put one cup in front of him.

"If for a moment I find it difficult, I will come back home. I promise I won't stress myself much," I said, looking into his eyes.

"Go, you stubborn girl and do well," his affirmative eyes blessed and showed care for me at the same moment.

I slumped into the prayer room to offer prayers before leaving the house. It's a cultivated habit to offer a prayer before leaving home, which my parents taught me.

"Dear God, I won't ask you to get me passing marks or an easy paper today. Just bless me with enormous strength for three long hours. Make me courageous enough to sit and write. As always, be with me."

Soon, a cab rode me to the destination. I learned that my exam would be conducted on the first floor of the building after checking my enrollment number on the list. The building had no escalator or elevator, so climbing stairs was a hurdle. Every step on the staircase was painful. Once I reached the room, the invigilator showed empathy and provided me with a question paper and answer sheet at the desk. She took my belongings and safely kept them aside.

All I remember afterward is that I continued writing till the bell rang. It was after a long time that I could sit for hours. I felt the pus ooze and dry up in these three hours. My lower clothes were stuck to my body because of the stickiness of pus. "Ahh," I uttered, as my eyes filled with tears. The invigilator, who came to hand over my belongings, put her hand on mine and said, "You are a strong woman; you will be fine soon, and I wish you the best for health and exams. If you can wait, I would like to accompany you outside."

It was a rare experience when an outsider touched my heart without being judgmental of my scary scars in recent times. This unconditional empathy toward each other makes the earth livable. Her slight gesture lit up a smile on my face. She held my hand and came out with me. She looked up for a cab and made sure that I had safely reached home.

I earned strength in myself and found that not everyone outside is cruel in this world. The world has generous people who can touch other people's hearts and be the best support system in life. The positive momentum of thoughts is much required to deal with bitter and sour situations in life. Time can flip, and life can be a worst nightmare, but time cannot make us losers until we believe in ourselves.

-Anonymous

Are You Fit?

written by Gene Frederic

Are you physically, emotionally and spiritually
fit?
Tell me all your shit,
Every bit.
Sit,
On it,
For a while.
What's your lifestyle,
Like?
Do you go on any hikes?
How often do you lose it,
And tell someone to go take a hike?
How often do you pray?
Stay,
Right there!
Don't go away.
Bare,
Your soup,
And heart.
Honesty with yourself is a start.
With who,
Or what,
Are you filling that hole,
In your heart?
So, I'm a Messianic Jew.
What are you?
What are you feeling in your gut,
Right now?
Ow!

Do you have faith in a God of any type?
Wipe,
Off your grin.
Honestly, do you realize the gravity of your
sins?
Does your resume get you in,
To Paradise?
Stop!
Don't spin the dice,
On your eternity.
Look at me as your spiritual cop.
Don't drop,
Dead,
Without making a decision.
This ain't no form of derision.
This is a heart to heart,
Plea.
You all need to realize,
That you need to be saved.
And you actually claim,
To be wise?!
This ain't no solitary blame,
Game.
You need to come out of your cave,
And wave,
The white,
Flag.
Stop your rebellious fight.
And, take that paper bag,
Off of your soul.
A lifestyle of unrepentant sin can take
its toll.

Jesus is ALL! you need.
I really don't care about how many
good deeds,
You've done,
Under the sun.
A need to be forgiven,
Is a battle that's been won.
Jesus bleeding on the cross,
Is a given.
Ultimately, your Boss,
Shall return.
Turn,
Or burn.
That's real.
It's a winnable deal.
It ain't based on how you feel.
Am I being,
Too hard,
On you?
I'd rather you be angry at me,
Then when you face your Creator and He,
tells you you've played the wrong cards.
True confession is freeing.
He'll is real,
Too.
It's all in your hands,
Where you go.
And, you can know,
For sure,
Where you go.
For Me,
The forgiveness offered by Jesus is the,

only cure.
I stand, on this being the only correct solution
There's too much unnecessary spiritual,
pollution.

Gene Frederic

Coming to terms with and letting go of the guilt and the shame that I felt because I felt all of these things were my fault. At 4 years old, logically, I knew it was not my fault that it happened, but I felt like I could have controlled the patterns that occurred afterward, and I didn't do a good job of that. Because I was supposed to make the world a better place, I wasn't expecting to be abused by my husband sexually, mentally, physically, or verbally. I wasn't expecting to start using drugs and alcohol. I wasn't supposed to lose a child at 23 and lose a relationship with my other child because I left my situation. I still cry and feel bad, but I have been able to slowly let go of things that were totally out of my control that happened. I have forgiven myself, and I have forgiven but not forgotten others for things that happened to me. I learned to show myself compassion, and the main thing is forgiveness and letting go of boating guilt and shame. It's only with therapy and my therapist that I have been able to overcome these things. Realized that I needed medication and I needed therapy as a maintenance program to maintain my mental health; I wasn't being a loser or a quitter because I had to take medicine, and I would get called crazy and psycho all the time. That's not true. Learning to be brave not only for myself but for others. Every day, I look for the positive, and I'm grateful for my life and everything in it.

- Pamela Perini

Hello, old friend...

We both know the importance of protecting our emotional, physical, and spiritual well-being. It's something we need to work on, though. In fact, I think it's something everyone needs to work on. I will start with the spiritual, the inside out, so to speak. When we talk about the spiritual, please know I'm talking about our spirit, not our beliefs or religion. What makes us similar and not what sets us apart. In fact, it focuses on how we're different and not the same, which is responsible for our spirits being damaged. We're too busy labeling everyone and everything rather than trying to find common ground. What difference does it make if we're black, white, Asian, straight, gay, lesbian, transgender, Christian, Jewish, atheist...you get where I'm coming from, don't you? If we remove the labels and start connecting at a spiritual level, it will change our spiritual well-being 100%. We will feel the human race's love, gratitude, and oneness. We will fill our souls with it. Still working from the inside out, we need to protect our emotional well-being.

We need to walk away from toxic people and toxic environments. Not easy, I know. Stick with me, and I'll explain. Toxicity directs us towards a negative, dangerous, and unhealthy way of behaving and reacting. I know you've felt it before. The tension, the anger, the frustration. It's like it's in the very air that we breathe. This is so damaging to our emotional well-being. It can even affect our physical well-being. But we'll get to that. These environments make you feel sad, unhappy, depressed, angry, frustrated. They can ruin your whole day if you let them. My suggestion to you, and you've experienced this yourself firsthand, is to remove yourself from these environments as much as possible. If work is toxic, request a transfer to another department. If the whole organization is toxic, find somewhere else to work. You can do this. No matter what anyone has told you. If it's a relationship, ask yourself, would I treat someone like this? If the answer is no, it may be time to step back or leave if it's a domestic situation. Scary huh? Anxiety producing? If you don't put yourself first, you can't help others you love and may need you. You can't pour from an empty cup, and you can't pour from a broken one, either. If it's a friendship that leaves you feeling horrible after a get-together or demeaned.

Undervalued, unimportant. Time to move on. And there's the physical. The inside and the outside. You can protect your physical self during sports by wearing a helmet, mouth guard, and elbow pads. You can protect yourself by wearing a seat belt in a car. You can protect yourself by eating correctly, having proper hygiene, and having regular check-ups with your doctor. You need to protect your spiritual and emotional well-being, too. There's a connection. And that connection can cause damage to any part if one part isn't protected. Stomach issues, issues with the heart, headaches, not eating enough or overeating, poor hygiene, and lack of sleep. These all need to be protected as well. I'm not saying any of this is easy. In fact, it can be challenging under certain circumstances. However, if we make a start, one step at a time, we will get there. And we will pave the way for understanding, acceptance, and love in future generations. You are worthy, you are loved, you matter.

Love and hugs,
Janet

- Janet D Sproule

I miei genitori, poco più che ventenni, sposati solo l'anno
precedente, trascorsero i nove mesi di gravidanza in felice attesa
del primo figlio. La gravidanza di mamma procedeva senza
difficoltà.

Il ginecologo di mia mamma la fece ricoverare nell'ospedale
giorni prima. Nessuno poteva immaginare quello che, di lì a
poco, sarebbe accaduto, sconvolgendo, letteralmente, tutta la mia
vita e di conseguenza mettendo a dura prova gli equilibri di una
giovane coppia.

Quel giorno il ginecologo, che aveva seguito mia mamma per
tutto il decorso della gravidanza, terminò il proprio turno nel
reparto.

A mia mamma le incominciarono le doglie; il tempo scorreva
inesorabilmente, i medici decisero, di fatto, di aspettare che gli
eventi si dipanassero da soli. Senza intervenire chirurgicamente.

Quando sono nato pesavo kg. 4,300, anche questo contribuì, e
non poco, all'aggravamento della situazione al momento della
mia venuta al mondo.

Fu questo lasso di tempo lasciato passare senza intervenire
chirurgicamente (senza, così, praticare un semplicissimo taglio
cesareo d'urgenza), unito ad un ultimo tentativo di rimediare in
extremis con l'ausilio del forcipe (strumento chirurgico a forma di
tenaglia) a causarmi un'interruzione dell'afflusso di ossigeno che
attraverso le arterie trasporta il sangue dal cuore affluisce al
cervello e viceversa. E di conseguenza venne

meno l'ossigenazione delle cellule celebrali causandomi un danno irreversibile. Danno, che in gergo medico, prodotto da un'asfissia prenatale.

Rimasi per parecchio tempo all'interno dell'incubatrice prenatale.
Nonostante tutto dopo sei mesi potei tornare a casa. Crescevo normalmente.

A sei mesi di età iniziai con la terapia occupazionale (è una disciplina riabilitativa che si occupa di aiutare le persone a svolgere le attività quotidiane necessarie per la vita indipendente), che ho continuato fino ai 16 anni di età; anni dopo, per breve periodo ho seguito un "corso" di linguaggio (che io volli abbandonare quasi subito); forse, visto con il senno di poi, avevo fatto meglio a continuarlo. Molto probabilmente mi sarebbe tornato utile nella pronuncia prima delle parole, e poi, nella costruzione di un discorso. Anche, e soprattutto, nel controllo del rispiro, tra una distonia (contrazione muscolare involontaria) e l'altra. A circa sei anni iniziai nuoto, che dopo, a 16 anni di età volli abbandonare; sono riuscito a nuotare "a dorso" con l'ausilio dei braccioli e delle pinne.

A cinque anni di età i miei genitori mi vollero iscrivere all'asilo pubblico, ma non nel paese dove abitavamo, ma nella città di Prato, con il corpo insegnante composto, non dalle suore, ma da maestre. Non avendo la possibilità di spostarmi da solo, non camminando, i miei genitori provarono con una sorta di macchina su cui stavo seduto e muovendo i piedi riuscivo a fare piccoli spostamenti.

Mamma a casa, intanto, si sforzava di volermi farmi imparare a leggere.

Un aneddoto di quel periodo dell'asilo: alcune volte una maestra, quando andava al bar per un caffè mi portava con lei. Era, così, l'unica occasione, per me, per sgranchirmi le gambe.
La difficoltà nell'imparare a leggere è stata quella che una volta letto, parte di una parola e arrivato in fondo non riuscivo a mettere assieme i singoli pezzi per farla diventare, poi, un'unica parola da pronunciare. E il saper leggere, anche poco, sembrava requisito indispensabile per accedere e potersi iscrivere alla prima classe elementare.

I miei genitori decisero che Mamma rimanesse, con me, a casa e che non lavorasse. Così, mamma, ogni giorno s'impegnava nel farmi imparare a leggere. Fin quando, sulla nostra strada si svelò, su un libro, la parola CAVALLO. Dapprima la sillabavo soltanto, arrivando in
fondo per dire la parola completa e non sapevo più ciò che avevo letto soltanto un attimo prima. Poi un giorno, a un tratto, arrivato in fondo alla parola, sillabandola come di solito, CA – VAL – LO provando a ripeterla unendo le sillabe; mia mamma, improvvisamente, sentì uscire delle mie labbra, con suo stupore, la parola CAVALLO – non più sillabata – ma leggevo la parola completa e, una volta finito di leggere sapevo il significato della parola appena letta. Fu il più importante scoglio superato che mi permise di accedere all'istruzione. E così potei frequentare le scuole elementari. Anche se ora si presentava un altro problema; quello di stare seduto cinque ore su di una sedia. Impossibile all'epoca per me; venne studiata dai miei genitori e fatta realizzare da un artigiano una poltrona con la struttura in legno e interamente imbottita, in più aveva anche un poggia

piedi. E lì trascorsi tutte le ore dei cinque anni delle scuole
elementari. Io non tenevo la penna in mano per scrivere; un
po' per i miei movimenti distonici, e un po' perché non adopravo
la mano destra. Allora provarono a sostituire la classica "penna"
per scrivere con una macchina da scrivere, elettronica, con
un'apposita tastiera, molto più grande, e piena di fori. Ogni foro
aveva al suo interno un tasto che corrispondeva alla giusta lettera
dell'alfabeto. E così potei scrivere i miei primi pensieri anch'io.
Chiaramente cercavo di essere il più conciso possibile per ridurre
al minimo il dispendio di energia, e di tempo. Procedimento
questo, che con il passare del tempo pensieri mi ha portato pian
piano ad essere coinciso anche nel parlato; mi accorsi che
risparmiavo energie, tempo e accrescevo la quantità espositiva
con l'ugual dispendio di energie, e quindi di affaticamento
fisico.

Nel frattempo, in estate, i miei genitori, su espresso consiglio
medico, cercavano di farmi trascorre il più tempo possibile al
mare. Principalmente per due motivi: in primis, per il
clima caldo-asciutto. Venne allora privilegiata la costa della
Versilia, sul mar Tirreno, caratterizzata per aver il mare con la
spiaggia di sabbia su un versante e sul versante opposto le
Alpi Apuane. Queste due caratteristiche creano un binomio per
avere un microclima caldo e asciutto; l'ideale per mettere in
pratica, quello che i medici, avevano consigliato ai mei genitori,
per me, come cura. Si trattava di pochi accorgimenti: agevolare,
in tutto e per tutto il bambino nel suo movimento del corpo e
creare appositamente stimoli, sempre nuovi. Altro lato, di vitale
importanza: socializzare. Anche se in quello non ho mai avuto
alcun tipo di problema grazie a tre delle mie caratteristiche: il
carattere calmo e tranquillo, gli occhi espressivi e il sorriso
sempre pronto a spuntare.

Fu proprio in questo contesto, vacanziero, che mamma e babbo misero in atto un vero e proprio piano. Il loro scopo era, come detto, di farmi fare movimento e allo stesso tempo di radunare, attorno a me, alcuni bambini per giocare insieme. E così fecero: durante la giornata, a turno, mamma e babbo giocarono assieme a me per coinvolgere altri bambini. La cosa più bella che i miei genitori si erano inventati per farmi fare movimento coinvolgendo gli altri bambini, era una specie di gara che consisteva nel percorrere tutto il tratto di spiaggia (partendo dalla battigia fino ad arrivare allo stabilimento balneare) in ginocchio. Così facendo mi rafforzavo i muscoli del corpo e aumentavo la dilatazione sia dei polmoni che della gabbia toracica. Forse è stato l'unico spazio temporale che mi ha più reso, e in cui mi sono sentito, più libero in tutta la mia vita.

Un'altra cosa che mi sorprese fu' quando la mia famiglia nel 1979, dopo anni che stava cercando un casale in campagna, come seconda casa, trovò un podere a Carmignano, in collina, tutto (rovinato) disabitato. Io avevo circa cinque anni di età. Arrivai con la mia famiglia al completo assieme ai nonni paterni che abitavano con noi. Mi presero in braccio e scendemmo. Scesi di macchina, quel posto fin ad ieri sconosciuto mi sembro subito casa; l'unico luogo in cui mi sembrava naturale vivere. Come l'avessi conosciuto da sempre, o meglio come se quel posto mi avesse chiamato. Da lì a poco decidemmo di tornarci ad abitare stabilmente in un'ala che ristrutturammo quasi subito.

Ristrutturammo immediatamente l'antica casa padronale e decidemmo di tornarci stabilmente. Io, nel frattempo, conclusi l'ultimo anno delle scuole elementari a Prato.

Nell'anno stesso mi iscrissero alle scuole medie del paese di Carmignano. Fu per me un po' traumatico perché mi trovai tutti i compagni di classe nuovi, mai conosciuti. Feci un passo avanti perché passai dalla mia poltrona imbottita con il poggia piedi, a riuscire a stare in posizione eretta con la schiena su una comunissima sedia di scuola. L'unica cosa che differenziava la mia sedia erano i braccioli. Mi permettevano di essere un po' più sicuro nel non cadere di lato.

Nel frattempo io continuavo come ancora oggi dopo tanti anni ad aver bisogno di aiuto di una terza persona per compiere ogni singola azione dal mattino, quando mi venivano a svegliare, fino a sera per andare a dormire. E tutt'ora, dopo cinquant'anni è ancora così.

Non cammino da solo, non mi porto il cibo alla bocca, non mi vesto da solo, non riesco a lavarmi nemmeno una mano in autonomia, non mi lavo i denti da solo; e non riesco nemmeno a essere indipendente quando ho una necessità fisiologica. Dipendo, in tutto e per tutto, per ogni comunissima e banalissima azione che miliardi di persone nel mondo
ogni singolo giorno possono fare in autonomia, da soli; senza dover sempre chiedere a un'altra persona l'aiuto per compiere ogni minima azione o gesto più o meno complesso di vitale importanza per la sopravvivenza di un essere umano.

Durante i tre anni delle scuole medie nel paese dove ci eravamo trasferiti a Carmignano, feci un primo incontro che mi cambiò, decisamente, la vita. Io continuavo, come alle scuole elementari, ad avere, in classe un'insegnante di sostegno. L'insegnante di sostegno che doveva aver il compito di prendermi i libri di testo, aprigli alla pagina che indicava il professore, sottolineare i passi più salienti e prendere appunti. Né più e né meno di quello che facevano i miei compagni di classe, alunni, di 14-15 anni di età. Mentre se, tutt'oggi, vado a prendere qualsiasi libro di testo, di quegli anni, trovo dei libri con delle pagine intonse, ingiallite dal tempo si, ma senza alcuna sottolineatura. I quaderni che dovrebbero essere pieni di appunti, delle varie materie, sono sostanzialmente inesistenti. A metà mattina, in classe, vi erano dieci minuti per fare merenda, l'insegnante di sostegno andava per i fatti suoi e io rimanevo in classe con la merenda nella cartella; menomale arrivava, quasi sempre, un addetto alle pulizie della scuola, che senza avere alcun compito nei miei confronti, di propria spontanea volontà, e gratuitamente, tutti giorni mi permetteva di fare colazione mettendomi a mia completa disposizione le proprie mani. Per evitare di dovermi fare dare bere con il classico bicchiere, escogitai un modo alternativo per poter bere in autonomia; infatti, incominciai a bere con l'ausilio di una semplice cannuccia.

Il secondo anno, nel 1987 circa, che frequentavo le scuole medie, ebbi la fortuna di incontrare un professore di matematica con una vera passione per l'informatica che si dedicò a me non solo nell'orario prettamente scolastico, ma impegnò del proprio tempo libero per trasmettermi le prime rudimentali nozioni per usare un computer. Quel professore inconsapevolmente, fin allora estraneo, mi stava facendo dono il poter finalmente scrivere per la mia prima volta, pur con un dito solo, in piena autonomia ogni mio pensiero. Realizzando, sul modello di quella che usavo già con la macchina da scrivere, appositamente per me, una tastiera tre volte più grande rispetto alla tastiera standard, e con la superficie pari, non con i tasti in rilievo, ma piena di fori; dentro a ciascun foro c'era la lettera. Potevo, con quella invenzione, appoggiare tranquillamente la mia mano sulla testiera senza che il peso della mia mano stessa andasse a sfiorare alcun tasto; per poi, con tutta calma andare a premere il tasto prescelto nel foro corrispondente. L'imparare a usare il computer fu provvidenziale per la mia vita. Un altro insegnamento importantissimo che il mio professore di matematica mi ha trasmesso e che mi è risultato fondamentale, è stato il consiglio per ricordare i vari comandi o le varie serie di comandi per poter eseguire quella o questa operazione con i diversi programmi; in pratica di non segnarmi niente, e andare a memoria. Dovevo, cioè, ricordarmi tutto ciò che mi era utile, facendo affidamento solo, ed esclusivamente, sulla mia memoria. Io di questo espediente né ho fatto un mantra; applicandolo a qualunque materia, mi è sempre stato utile. Con il mio professore di matematica, con il quale passavo del tempo, nacque una bella amicizia (tan tè che per un periodo, quando aveva del tempo libero); veniva a prendermi in classe chiedendo il permesso al professore di turno, e mi portava nella palestra della scuola dove mi faceva provare a camminare da solo, fare due o tre passi per volta. Ahimè, in questo, non ci siamo riusciti. Da tutto ciò è rimasto il sapere usare il computer, e successivamente, internet con tutte le sue applicazioni, oltre ad una fortissima amicizia che dura ancora oggi.

Nel 1988, in piena estate, nel mese di luglio, approfittando del periodo di ferie scolastico, i miei genitori decisero di usufruire proprio di quella mia pausa dagli studi per farmi affrontare un intervento chirurgico, non più procrastinabile. Si trattava di andare a fare tre interventi chirurgici per ciascuna gamba: attraverso piccole incisioni a forma di coda di rondine con i bisturi sui tendini, sarebbero diventati più lunghi e permettendomi di nuovo, di riappoggiare il tallone del piede a terra durante il passo. Rimasi perciò per tutto il mese di luglio con

i gessi a entrambe le gambe (da cima a fondo compreso i piedi).
Trascorsi i miei trenta giorni con tutte e due le gambe ingessate a
casa e quel tempo caldo continuava a farsi sentire sotto il gesso la
pelle iniziava a prudere insistentemente, non mi potevo muovere.
Contavo i giorni che mi separavano dal togliermi i gessi.
Nessuno mi aveva detto ciò che mi attendeva una volta tagliato il
gesso. Le mie gambe erano rimaste chiuse e immobili per 30
lunghi giorni e ciò aveva provocato una marcata diminuzione
della muscolatura, quasi inesistente in quel momento, oltre alla
sensibilità accentuata; il semplice sfioramento della pelle
delle gambe con una leggera spazzola per neonati mi procurava
dolore. La cosa più dolorosa si realizzò quando, al momento
dell'apertura dei gessi le ginocchia improvvisamente si piegavano
di scatto. Il dolore era fortissimo e acuto. Con l'aiuto della mia
fisioterapista riuscii ad archiviare anche quella bruttissima
esperienza. L'unica nota positiva della vicenda era che avevo
risolto per sempre, il problema legato al mio modo sbagliato di
appoggiare il piede a terra. Ora non appoggiavo più in punta il
piede, ma avevo ripreso l'andatura normale del passo andando a
poggiare tutta la pianta del piede a terra.

Mi consigliarono, terminate le scuole medie nel giugno del 1989,
un istituto tecnico commerciale lontanissimo da casa. Distava
venti chilometri da dove abitavamo noi. La scelta di quella
scuola, così distante da casa, era stata dettata dalla certezza di
trovare un computer in classe a mia completa disposizione e un
corpo docente che doveva essere già "allenato" a trattare con
alunni portatori di handicap.

Tutte queste "belle" certezze vennero spazzate via non appena
entrai il primo giorno in classe. Il computer che doveva essere in
classe sin dal primo giorno di scuola non c'era, e non arrivò in

tutti i cinque o sei anni delle mie scuole superiori. Quella parte di docenti "allenati" a trattare con alunni con handicap aveva chiesto e ottenuto il trasferimento. Io mi ritrovai in una classe con il corpo docente totalmente ostile verso ogni tipo di handicap e senza alcun computer.

Nel passaggio dalle scuole medie alle scuole superiori era cambiato anche il tipo di assistenza in classe e io mi ritrovai, dall'avere l'insegnante di sostegno ad avere un assistente non preparato per il ruolo che era chiamato a svolgere. Non che fossero necessari requisiti particolarmente complessi per il reclutamento; in quel momento l'unico requisito, davvero essenziale, era quello di trovare una persona empatica: una persona che avesse avuto la curiosità di conoscermi, di capire quali erano le mie effettive necessità. Eppure tutt'ora io mi soffermo a riflettere su quello che è stato: mi chiedo come una qualsiasi persona possa aver tenuto un tale comportamento verso un altro essere umano, che per giunta era impossibilitato, come ero io, a reagire. Non era sempre lo stesso assistente, si avvicendavano diverse persone durante tutto l'anno scolastico. Più tardi mi imbattei in un individuo che mi rese la vita più complicata del mio solito.

Io che per la mia invalidità non ero in grado di fare nessuna di quelle azioni tipiche per uno studente qualunque, come prendere il libro o il quaderno dalla cartella, né tenere aperto il libro di testo aperto sul banco, e ben che meno, di prendere alcun tipo di appunto. Non reggevo nemmeno la penna in mano. Quando mi ritrovai iscritto alle scuole superiori, e più precisamente all'istituto tecnico commerciale "Piero Calamandrei" per ragionieri e periti commerciali, si ripropose, insistentemente il problema di come farmi svolgere i compiti pomeridiani a casa per il giorno successivo. I miei genitori pensando ad una soluzione si ricordarono di quando, due anni prima (in seconda media) ebbi bisogno di alcune ripetizioni nel mese di luglio. Mia mamma, allora, telefonò alla persona che mi fece le ripetizioni e la incontrò: le disse, che io avevo iniziato da poco la prima classe della scuola superiore e che avevo bisogno di un aiuto giornaliero per svolgere i compiti a casa. E così si accordarono: dal giorno seguente mi avrebbe dato lezioni private, dietro compenso, per due ore del proprio tempo, al giorno per potermi aiutare a svolgere i compiti. Conoscendola meglio quella ragazza con gli occhiali, scoprii che aveva una vera e propria passione per la letteratura, era una vera divoratrice di libri e quella passione è riuscita a trasmettermela; non la ringrazierò mai abbastanza per avermi trasmesso la passione per la lettura e per lo studiare. Questa collaborazione si protrasse fino alla quinta delle scuole superiori con il mio primo vero traguardo, il diploma.

Una mia intuizione che con il tempo si rilevò di fondamentale importanza e che mi cambiò in meglio il trascorrere tutte quelle ore di scuola sempre seduto, senza nemmeno muovermi, fu il cambiare sedia. Mi venne l'idea di portarmi da casa una semplice sedia da ufficio; quelle con le cinque ruotine; mi permise di spostarmi pur rimanendo seduto. Quell'idea fu di fondamentale importanza: ora, con quella sedia da ufficio potevo muovermi, anche spostarmi sotto il banco di scuola, mi sembrò un grandissimo passo verso l'autonomia che avevo sempre teso. In quel momento grazie a quell'escamotage, almeno nell'intervallo, potevo finalmente uscire di classe e come avevo sempre visto fare a tutti i miei compagni delle scuole elementari, medie, e superiori. Fu una bella sensazione di libertà. E così proseguii nelle scuole superiori.

In quarta superiore ebbi il mio terzo incontro che cambiò, una volta ancora, il mio percorso di vita. Nell'indirizzo di studi di ragioneria era contemplata la materia "diritto" ed ebbi la fortuna di trovare una professoressa che non insegnava solamente la materia, ma insegnava con la passione dello studioso. Si percepivano le spiegazioni e non si trattava più di una semplice materia scolastica. Ma c'era di più. Io fino ad allora avevo avuto un distacco totale tra quello che studiavo e i miei veri interessi (come la lettura, la musica, l'arte e il teatro). Questo incontro mi fu, certamente, provvidenziale. Mi affascinai talmente tanto alla materia del diritto che una volta diplomato, fu quasi sequenziale per me scegliere giurisprudenza come facoltà universitaria. Intuii, fortunatamente per me, che i disagi delle persone con handicap avevano, tutti, un'unica matrice, che si poteva benissimo rintracciare nella legge. Contrariamente a ciò che pensavano i miei genitori non mi volli fermare con gli studi al diploma.

Iscritto alla facoltà di giurisprudenza dell'università di Firenze presi una decisione; anche se confesso che sul momento sembrò a tutti una pazzia, ma ancora una volta la mia "vocina" si fece sentire; mi susurrava "più libertà" e io a quel punto decisi lasciarmi guidare. Decisi di abbondonare tutte le mie "confort zone" e scelsi di fare un salto nel buio: l'insegnante a casa per i compiti decisi che non mi fosse più necessaria e che da lì in poi quello che sarei riuscito a fare sarebbe dipeso solo da me. L'uso del mio "amato" computer che mi aveva donato tanto tempo prima più "libertà", era ora diventato una zavorra che mi tratteneva. Io, in quel momento, non avevo bisogno di essere trattenuto da niente e nessuno. Così, liberato da lacci e lacciuoli, iniziai con il prendere pian piano coscienza del percorso di studi che si prospettava davanti a me. Si trattava di un corso di laurea,

giurisprudenza, con ventiquattro esami totali. Iniziai allora a
frequentare la facoltà e le lezioni in aula. Ben presto, mi
resi conto che frequentare in aula le lezioni per me era troppo
stancante fisicamente. I vari dipartimenti erano dislocati per tutto
il centro storico di Firenze, lo stesso centro storico quello di
Firenze con molte aree interdette al transito delle auto e con
pochissimi parcheggi. Allora, modificai, ulteriormente il mio
progetto di studi universitari che così mi ero immaginato fosse
essere quello dell'assidua frequentazione delle varie lezioni dei
corsi che volevo seguire. Muovermi per me con la sedia a rotelle
diventava sempre più difficoltoso: non era migliorato il muoversi
all'interno delle varie strutture che erano manchevoli di
tutte quelle infrastrutture per l'accesso di una carrozzina per
portatori di handicap. Allora, decisi di studiare da casa; da lì in
poi, avrei "fatto" l'università da non frequentante. E così
feci. L'ostacolo più grande fu quando arrivai a dover prendere
appunti con la penna in mano; lo so che, per la maggior parte
delle persone è la cosa più "normale" di questo mondo, ma
non per me. All''inizio non tenevo nemmeno la penna in mano.
C'era un problema che andava analizzato con calma se si voleva
trovare una soluzione. Le braccia e le mani
risultavano inutilizzabili. A questo punto andai a ricercare ciò
che adesso chiamano le capacità residue, lo feci da solo e ignaro
di cosa fosse e di dove dover cercare. Mi dissi che per fare una
cosa o un'azione forse esisteva anche un altro modo, già, però
questi altri modi andavano scoperti provando e riprovano
andando per tentativi.

Sceglievo l'esame e andavo a parlare con il professore della
materia; mi presentavo con tutte le mie difficoltà, mi facevo dire
i titoli dei libri di testo e acquistavo i libri. A questo punto mi
prendevo tutto il tempo necessario per sottolineare con la mano

43

sinistra a lapis. Il tratto della mia sottolineatura non era una linea uniforme, ma composto da minuscoli trattini più o meno storti che uniti tutti assieme componevano un'unica linea.

Nel 2001, dopo aver sostenuto nove esami universitari, fui costretto, letteralmente, ad abbondonare i miei amati studi per problemi di salute. Il mio "corpo" mi poneva davanti ad un out out; mi dovetti fermare per curarmi corpo e mente, come dicevano gli antichi romani mens sana in corpore sano. E io, anche se a malincuore, mi dovetti fermare. Mi fermai ben cinque, lunghi anni per curarmi; senza alcuna certezza se e quando avrai potuto riprendere i miei amati studi. Nel periodo che fui costretto ad abbandonare i miei studi per curarmi rimasi a casa tra una lettura di un buon libro e l'ascolto di un disco e volli sperimentare il disegno a mano libera. Presi coscienza, da subito, che realizzare un disegno con una sola linea era per me impossibile. Pensai allora ad un modo alternativo che mi avesse permesso di raggiungere l'obiettivo di poter disegnare. Elaborai un metodo partendo proprio dal come io sottolineavo i libri di testo universitari: non con un'unica linea di lapis, ma mettendo un trattino, più o meno storto accanto all'altro così da costruire con piccoli trattini storti una sola riga. Così facendo potei disegnare anche io. Una volta ancora mi ero messo alla prova per vedere dove si poteva alzare per me l'asticella delle mie potenzialità. Riuscii anche se molto imprecisamente, nel mio intento di disegnare.

Per fortuna mia riuscii a ristabilirmi e tentare di riniziare a pensare di riprendere i miei amati studi, da dove ero stato costretto a interrompergli. Con mia grande gioia, nell'aprile del 2014, mi laureai in giurisprudenza scrivendo tutta la tesi di laurea con il "solo" ausilio di un "vecchio" portatile. Riuscii, con mia grande sorpresa a discutere, oralmente, nell'intera tesi; malgrado il mio linguaggio disarticolato. Mi sembrò, per un attimo, di "toccare" il cielo con un dito.

-Paolo Lastrucci

My parents, just over twenty, who were married only the year before, spent the nine months of pregnancy happily awaiting their first child. Mom's pregnancy was progressing without difficulties. My mom's gynecologist had her admitted to the hospital days before. No one could imagine what was about to happen, literally shaking up my entire life and, consequently, putting a strain on the balance of a young couple's marriage.

That day, the gynecologist, who had followed my mom throughout the course of the pregnancy, finished his shift in the ward.

My mom started having contractions; time was passing inexorably, and the doctors decided to wait for events to unfold on their own without intervening surgically. I weighed 4.300 kg (over nine pounds) when I was born. This also greatly contributed to the worsening of the situation at the time of my arrival in the world.

It was this period of time left to pass without surgical intervention (without, thus, performing a very simple emergency cesarean section), combined with a final attempt to remedy at the last minute with the help of forceps (a surgical instrument shaped like tongs) to cause an interruption of the oxygen flow that carries blood from the heart to the brain and vice versa. And consequently, the oxygenation of the brain cells was lacking, causing me irreversible damage. Damage, which in medical jargon was caused by "prenatal asphyxia."

I remained in the neonatal incubator for quite some time. Despite everything, after six months, I was able to return home. I was growing normally.

At six months old, I started occupational therapy (it is a rehabilitative discipline that focuses on helping people perform activities of daily living), which I continued until I was 16 years old. Years later, for a short period, I took a "course" in language (which I wanted to abandon almost immediately); perhaps, in hindsight, I would have been better to continue it. Most likely, it would have been useful to me to aid me in the pronunciation of syllables and then in constructing a speech. Also, especially in controlling my breath, between one dystonia (involuntary muscle contraction) and the other. At about six years old, I started swimming, which, later, at 16 years old, I wanted to stop. I managed to swim "on my back" with the help of arm floats and fins.

At five years old, my parents wanted to enroll me in a public kindergarten, not in the town where we lived, but in the city of Prato, with the teaching staff was made up of teachers, not nuns. Not having the ability to move by myself, or walking, my parents put together a machine that I could sit on, and by moving my feet, I could make small movements.

Mom at home, meanwhile, was trying to make me learn to read.

An anecdote from that kindergarten period: sometimes, a teacher, when she went to the bar for a coffee, would take me with her. This was the only opportunity for me to stretch my legs.

The difficulty in learning to read was that once I read part of a word and got to the end, I couldn't put the individual pieces together to make it become a word to pronounce. Knowing how to read, even a little, seemed essential to access and enroll in the first grade of elementary school.

My parents decided that Mom would stay home with me and not work. So, Mom, every day, committed to making me learn to read. Until, one day, the word HORSE (CAVALLO in Italian) revealed itself in a book. At first, I only syllabicated it, getting to the bottom to say the complete word, and I no longer knew what I had read. Then one day, suddenly, having reached the end of the word, syllabicating as usual, CA-VAL-LO trying to repeat it by joining the syllables; my Mom suddenly heard come out of my lips, to her surprise, the word CAVALLO. No longer syllabicated- but I read the complete word and, once I finished reading, I knew the meaning of the word I just read. It was the most important hurdle I overcame, allowing me to access education. And so I was able to attend elementary school. However, another problem arose: sitting for five hours on a chair, which was impossible for me at that time. My parents brainstormed and came up with the idea for a chair, which they then had made by a craftsman. The chair was wooden, fully padded, and had a footrest. There, I spent all the hours of the five years of elementary school. I did not hold the pen in my hand to write, partially because I did not use my right hand. Then they tried to replace the classic "pen" for writing with an electronic typewriter, with a special larger keyboard with holes. Each hole had a key corresponding to the correct letter of the alphabet. And so, I was able to write my first thoughts. I tried to be as concise as possible to minimize energy expenditure and time. This process, which gradually led me to be concise even in speech, made me realize that I was saving energy and time and increasing the amount of exposition with the same energy expenditure, and therefore physical fatigue.

In the meantime, in summer, my parents, following the medical advice of my doctors, allowed me to spend as much time as possible at sea, mainly, for the warm-dry climate. The coast of Versilia, on the Tyrrhenian Sea, was favored, characterized by the sea with the sandy beach on one side and the Apuan Alps on the other side.

This rehabilitation plan centered on a few adjustments: to facilitate the child's body movement in every way and to create new stimuli. Another aspect of vital importance was socialization. Even though I never had any problem with this, thanks to three of my characteristics: my calm and quiet character, my expression, and my smile, which was always ready to make an appearance.

Mom and Dad implemented a real and proper plan in this vacation context. Their goal was, as mentioned, to get me to move and, simultaneously, to gather other children around me to play together. And so, they did. During the day, Mom and Dad played with me to involve other children.

The most beautiful thing my parents had come up with to get me to move while involving the other children was a race that covered the entire stretch of beach (starting from the water's edge to reach the beach establishment) on my knees. In doing so, I strengthened muscles and increased the expansion of both the lungs and the rib cage. Perhaps it was the only space/time continuum that allowed me to feel the freest I had in my entire life thus far.

Another surprising and synchronistic occurrence happened in 1979, when, after years of looking for a farmhouse in the countryside as a second home, my family found an uninhabited, demolished farmhouse in the hills of Carmigano. I was about five years old. I arrived with my family, including my paternal grandparents, who lived with us. They picked me up, and we got out of the car; that place – unknown until yesterday, immediately felt like home, the only place where it felt natural to live. As if I had known it forever, or better, yes, as if that place had called me. Shortly after, we decided to return to live permanently in a wing that we renovated almost immediately.

We restored the old manor house and decided to return to it permanently. In the meantime, I completed my last year of elementary school in Prato.

In the same year, I was enrolled in the middle school in Carmigano. It was a bit traumatic because I had completely new classmates and did not know anyone. I stepped forward from my cushioned armchair with a footrest to sitting upright with my back on a standard school chair. The only thing that differentiated my chair was the armrests. They allowed me to be a bit more secure to avoid falling off the side.

In the meantime, I continued, as I still do today after so many years, to need help from another person to perform every single action from the morning, when they came to wake me up, until evening, when I went to sleep. And even now, after fifty years, it is still so.

I cannot walk alone, I cannot bring food to my mouth, I do not dress myself, I cannot wash even one hand independently. I do not brush my teeth alone, and I cannot even be independent while going to the bathroom. I depend on someone else for anything and everything. This includes every small and trivial action that billions of people can do independently, every day, without always having to ask another person for help.

During the three years of middle school in the town where we had moved to Carmignano, I had an encounter that changed my life. I continued to have a support teacher in class. The support teacher was supposed to take my textbooks, open them to the page indicated by the teacher, underline the most important passages, and take notes. No more and no less than what my classmates, students aged 14-15 years old, did. When I look at any textbook from those years, I find books with untouched pages, yellowed by time, but without any underlining. The notebooks that should be full of notes from various subjects are essentially non-existent. In the middle of the morning, there were ten minutes for a snack in class. The support teacher went about her own business, and I stayed in class with my snack in my bag; luckily, almost always, a school janitor, who had no obligation or responsibility toward me every day, allowed me to have breakfast by lending me his hands. I even devised an alternative way to drink independently; I started drinking with the help of a simple straw.

In the second year, around 1987, when I was attending middle school, I had the good fortune to meet a math teacher with a true passion for computer science who worked with me during school hours and his own time. He taught me, free of charge, how to use a computer. Until then, that teacher was a complete stranger, unbeknownst to me, giving me the gift of finally being able to write for the first time, even with just one finger, fully autonomously, every thought of mine. Based on the model of what I already used with the typewriter, specifically for me, a keyboard three times larger than the standard keyboard, and with a flat surface, not with raised keys, but full of holes; inside each hole was a letter. With that invention, I could comfortably rest my hand on the keyboard without the weight of my hand touching any key and then calmly press the chosen key in the corresponding hole. Learning to use the computer was providential for my life. Another vital lesson that my math teacher passed on to me and that was fundamental for me, was the advice to remember the various commands to perform this or that operation in different programs; basically, not to write anything down, but to remember everything useful to me, relying only on my memory.

I have made a mantra of this trick; applying it to any subject has always been helpful. With my math teacher, with whom I spent time, a beautiful friendship was born (so much so that for a period when he had free time); he would come to pick me up in class asking for permission from the teacher on duty, and he would take me to the school gym where he made me try to walk on my own, take two or three steps at a time. Alas, in this, we failed.

From all this, I learned to use the computer and, later, the internet with all its applications, in addition to a very strong friendship that still lasts today.

In 1988, in the middle of summer, in July, taking advantage of the school holiday period, my parents decided to take advantage of that break from my studies to have me undergo a surgical procedure that was no longer postponable. It involved three surgeries for each leg: through small incisions shaped like a swallowtail with the scalpel on the tendons, they would become longer and allow me again to rest the heel of my foot on the ground while walking. Therefore, I stayed for the entire month of July with casts on both legs (from top to bottom, including the feet). I spent my thirty days with both legs in casts at home, and that hot weather continued to be felt under the cast, and my skin began to itch insistently; I couldn't move. I counted the days that separated me from having my casts removed. No one had told me what awaited me once the cast was cut. My legs had been closed and immobile for 30 long days, and this had caused a marked decrease in muscle mass, which was almost nonexistent. At that moment, in addition to heightened sensitivity, the simple touch of the skin of the legs with a light baby brush caused me pain. The most painful thing happened after removing the casts. My knees suddenly bent sharply. The pain was extreme and sharp. With the help of my physiotherapist, I managed to archive that horrible experience as well. The only positive note of the affair was that I had permanently solved the problem related to my wrong way of placing my foot on the ground. Now, I no longer put my foot on tiptoe, but I had resumed the step's normal gait by placing the sole of my foot on the ground.

After finishing middle school in June 1989, they advised me to go to a technical institute that was very far from home. It was twenty kilometers away from where we lived. The choice of that school, so far from home, was dictated by the certainty of finding a computer in class at my complete disposal and a teaching staff that was supposed to be already "trained" to deal with students with disabilities.

All these "nice" certainties were swept away as soon as I entered the first day of class. The computer that was supposed to be in class from the first day of school was not there and did not arrive in all five or six years of my high school. That part of the teachers "trained" to deal with students with disabilities had requested and obtained a transfer. I found myself in a class with a teaching staff totally hostile to any type of disability and without any computer.

In the transition from middle school to high school, the type of assistance in class changed, and I found myself from having a support teacher to having an unprepared assistant for the role he was called to perform. Not that there were particularly complex requirements necessary for recruitment; at that moment, the only essential requirement was to find an empathetic person who would have had the curiosity to get to know me and understand my actual needs. And yet I still pause to reflect on what has been: I wonder how any person could have behaved in such a way towards another human being who was also unable, as I was, to react. It was not always the same assistant; different people took turns throughout the school year. Later, I encountered an individual who made my life more complicated than usual.

Due to my disability, I could not perform typical actions of a regular student, like taking the book or notebook from the backpack, keeping the textbook open on the desk, and much less taking notes. I did not even hold a pen in my hand. When I enrolled in high school, specifically at the technical, commercial institute "Piero Calamandrei" for accountants and expert commercials,

54

the problem of how to get me to do the homework arose again. Thinking of a solution, my parents remembered when, two years earlier (in the second year of middle school), I needed some tutoring in July. My mom then called the person who tutored me and met her: she told her that I had just started the first year of high school and needed daily help to do my homework at home. And so, they agreed: from the following day, she would give me private lessons, for a fee, for two hours of her own time a day to help me with my homework. Getting to know her better, that girl with glasses, I discovered that she had a true passion for literature. She was a true bookworm, and that passion was passed on to me; I will never thank her enough for instilling a love in myself for reading and studying. This collaboration lasted until the fifth year of high school with my first real milestone, the diploma.

An intuition that over time proved to be of fundamental importance and changed me for the better, while passing long hours of school, always sitting, without even moving, was that I change my chair. I had the idea to bring a simple office chair from home, one with five wheels that allowed me to move while remaining seated. That idea was of fundamental importance: now, with that office chair, I could move; even moving under the school desk felt like a huge step towards the autonomy I had always aimed for. Thanks to that trick, at least during the break, I could finally leave the classroom and do as I had always seen all my classmates do in elementary, middle, and high school. It was a nice feeling of freedom. And so, I continued in high school.

In my fourth year of high school, I had my third encounter that changed, once again, my path in life. In the accounting study program, the subject of "law" was included, and I was fortunate to find a teacher who not only taught the subject but taught with the passion of a scholar. The explanations were perceptible, and it was no longer just a simple school subject. But there was more. Until then, I had a total detachment between what I studied and my true interests (like reading, music, art, and theater). This encounter was certainly providential for me. I became so fascinated by the subject of law that once I graduated, it was almost sequential for me to choose law as my university faculty. I intuitively realized, fortunately for me, that the difficulties of people with disabilities all had a single root, which could easily be traced back in the law. Contrary to what my parents thought, I did not want to stop my studies at the diploma.

Enrolled in the law faculty at the University of Florence, I made a decision; even though I confess that at the moment it seemed crazy to everyone, once again my "little voice" made itself heard; it whispered to me "more freedom," and at that point, I decided to let myself be guided. I abandoned all my "comfort zones" and took a leap into the dark: the home tutor for homework; I decided I no longer needed it and that from then on, what I could do would depend only on me. Using my "beloved" computer, which had been given me so long ago, that used to provide more "freedom," was now a burden that held me back. At that moment, I did not need to be held back by anything or anyone. So, I freed myself from ties and snares, I gradually became aware of the study path ahead of me. It was a degree course in law, with twenty-four total exams. I then started attending the faculty and the classes in the classroom. Soon, I realized that attending classes in the classroom at the school was too physically exhausting for me. The various departments were scattered throughout the historic center of Florence, which is the same historic center of Florence, with many areas restricted to car traffic and very few parking spaces. So, I modified my university study plan to include the various courses I had imagined regularly attending, including the multiple lessons of the courses I wanted to follow. Moving around in a wheelchair was becoming increasingly difficult for me: it had not improved moving within the various structures that were lacking all those infrastructures for wheelchair access for people with disabilities. So, I decided to study from home; from then on, I would "do" university as a non-attending student. And so, I did.

The biggest obstacle was when I had to take notes with a pen in hand; I know that, for most people, it is the most "normal" thing in the world, but not for me. At first, I couldn't even hold the pen in my hand. There was a problem that needed to be analyzed calmly if one wanted to find a solution. My arms and hands were useless. At this point, I researched what is now called residual abilities; I did it alone and was unaware of what it was and where to look. I told myself that to do something or an action, there might be another way, yes, but these other ways had to be discovered by trying and retrying through attempts.

I would choose the exam and talk to the professor about the subject; I would present myself with all my difficulties; I would ask for the titles of the textbooks and buy the books. At this point, I would take all the time necessary to underline with my left hand using a pencil. The stroke of my underlining was not a uniform line but made up of tiny dashes that were less crooked that, when combined, formed a single line.

In 2001, after taking nine university exams, I was literally forced to abandon my beloved studies due to health problems. My "body" forced me to stop and to care of my body and mind, as the ancient Romans said, *"mens sana in corpore sano."* And I, although reluctantly, had to stop. I stopped for as long as five long years to care for myself without any certainty if and when I could resume my beloved studies. When I was forced to abandon my studies to take care of myself, I stayed at home. Between reading a good book and listening to a record; I wanted to experiment with freehand drawing. I immediately realized that creating a drawing with a single line was impossible. I then thought of an alternative way that would allow me to achieve the goal of being able to draw. I developed a method starting precisely from how I underlined university textbooks: not with a single pencil line, but by putting a dash, more or less crooked, next to the other to build with small crooked dashes a single line. In doing so, I could draw, too. Once again, I had put myself to the test to see where I could raise the bar of my potential. I succeeded, even though very imprecisely, in my attempt to draw.

Fortunately, I managed to recover and try to start thinking about resuming my beloved studies, from where I had been forced to interrupt them. To my great joy, in April 2014, I graduated in law, writing the entire thesis with the "only" aid of an "old" laptop. To my great surprise, I could discuss the whole thesis orally despite my disjointed language. For a moment, it seemed that I was "touching" the sky with my finger.

-Paolo Lastrucci

To myself. I want you to know that you are smart, kind, loving, generous, and funny, and you touch the hearts of every person you meet. You are strong. However, you will face lots of challenges, and you will overcome them. Don't be afraid to ask for help; this is a strength, not a weakness. There will be times when you feel like you can't go on anymore and like giving up. You will feel like you are alone. This is not true; it is just a feeling. You will sometimes feel that nobody knows or understands what you are going through. This is true as your experience is yours and yours alone. How you perceive it is based on everything you believe and all your experiences up until now. This is not to say that others do not experience similar hurt, heartache, or grief. Of course, they do. Talk as it helps.

One really good friend can make a huge difference. Be gentle with yourself; give yourself time to process things. You will lose people you love, and it will feel like they took your heart with them. It will feel surreal. The shock will cause sleepless nights, nightmares, and anxiety, and you just want to stop hurting. You will feel that you have no other option than to leave this life even though you don't want to. You will feel so disconnected from yourself, your family, your friends, absolutely everyone, and everything. You will feel guilt and shame and that it is somehow your fault. You will feel so angry that you don't even recognize yourself. All the 'What ifs" will start going around in your head. You will feel undeserving of being here. It will be so hard; you must find strength and fight back.

Fight for your life, fight for control, fight to stay; this will be your biggest challenge. You must never give up! You can't. Your family needs you. Your friends need you. You are here for a reason. You are so loved. You will get through this; you are a

60

warrior. Your losses have changed you forever and made you the strongest, most compassionate version of yourself. You will have a much better understanding of life and death. You are no longer afraid of death and realize the importance of living a beautiful life to the fullest. One that is full of love, joy, and happiness and understands its duality. When you love, you will also experience loss. I believe spirit is always with us; there is only love, and the fear we feel is the absence of love.

-Lisa Powell

Hello, I want to introduce myself. My name is Singha. Today, I will talk about emotional, physical, and spiritual well-being. As time passed, I realized that all these three things are the strongest pillars of human life. Everyone is connected with others. Here, I want to say that spiritual awakening balances the two aspects of our life. If we can balance our spiritual energy, it will also balance our physical and emotional energy. I was damaged, and I was an alcoholic person when I was in my twenties. I had a rough childhood, and I was going through that trauma in my teenage days. I was going through depression and anxiety issues, but by the grace of God, I was fortunate to meet my spiritual guru or teacher when I was around 27, and he completely changed my life. I use My spiritual energy to transform myself and cure all my traumas.

So, I suggest all of you reading this to connect with your spiritual energy and transform your life completely.

Lots of love and blessings,

-Singha

To Whom It May Concern:

This series contains multiple letters I've written to myself. In this one, I'm writing to you about the importance of my spirituality. Discovering my spiritual path was so vital to me that it's no overstatement to say it saved me.

Like many people, I grew up in the Christian religion. Being brought up in a religion is about social pressure. I do not believe it is wrong to bring children up in a religion of any kind. Religion gives people a moral foundation. A Sociology teacher of mine once said, "If God did not exist, we would have to invent him." If you are looking for a letter to tell you how to denounce religion, this is not it.

I love the teachings of Jesus Christ. I believe he is my savior. Without Jesus, I would have become a very - and I mean this in a deeply profound way - very bad person. I may have even killed myself without Jesus. I was close to becoming a bad person with Jesus in my life, but that is a letter for another time. I do not believe Christianity is the only path to spiritual health. I believe that God/Goddess is beyond our comprehension. It does not matter what path you take as long as you take one. That is what this letter is about.

As a child of a true narcissist, I was not allowed to be myself and was considered rebellious, sinful, and detestable. In reality, I was hurt, hidden, and angry. I went to church every Sunday because it made my parents look good. I sat with the family that was torturing me. I listened to how God loved me so much that he let his son die for me, and I was unworthy of such a sacrifice. I prayed to the same God they prayed to. I even believed the same way my family thought. I felt I was going to hell if I did not walk the walk and talk the talk. More than anything, I knew I was unworthy of existence. I believed that so much I was terrified to read my bible. I slept with it under my pillow, but I never read it. I never knew what it said.

That is a thing about religion. Many of us believe in the religion that is taught to us. We don't learn for ourselves what our faith is really about. Let that sink in for a few minutes if you grew up in a religion. Do you know if what you were taught to believe is what you should believe? Is it something that God/Goddess wishes you to believe? Do you understand it on a truly soulful and spiritual level?

The first step on my journey out of religion and into faith was a scary, rebellious one against my family. It was a question. If God was real, then God existed before Christianity. If God is real, God existed before man. There would be evidence somewhere, right? Even then, I loved Sociology.

I began to seek God out. I peeked out of my hidden hole and looked for God. The first time I read my bible, I thought I would burn up right then. I was gonna die. There was no way I was worthy enough to read the Word!

On top of that, I was questioning what I had been taught. I did not respect my parents, which was the strongest commandment in our home. I was going to hell, but at least I would have some answers.

I began to seek more and more as I grew up. One answer led to five more questions. Five more answers led to knowledge. Knowledge led to upset and hurt. My mother once told me I was a demon of the end times because 'I knew too much.' This was during a three-hour yelling session to beat into me why what I was doing set me personally against her. My brother asked me once, "Why do you want to know that?" He wanted me to just be ok with things as they were. I was told many times, "You need God, girl." Well, duh, I was looking for him, wasn't I? At one point, my parents put me in a mental ward. Granted, there was a lot of other stuff happening during all this, and I probably was a classic basket case.

Jesus said the truth will set you free. They killed him. Often, we, as a species, kill the truth. We torture and dismiss people who teach us the truth. As a species, we don't want people to look for truth. They are harder to control. We want them to toe the line. We want them to stay where they belong. Truth is a harsh mistress. It can get you killed. It was one of the first lessons I learned from the Jesus dude. That is a serious warning. Following a spiritual truth can and will make you different. Biology despises difference even if evolution helps survival. For better or worse, the human species is biological.

Many times on my journey, I was pretty sure I was insane. I was even accused of being a Witch more than once. Luckily, people don't openly burn witches anymore.

Through it all, Jesus taught me. God/Goddess taught me. I learned who I was. I learned I was not who I was taught to be. I was fearsomely created by a being so beyond the scope of my reasoning it was insane to touch the air it passed through.

I am fifty-five years old now. I still do not know the answers. I do believe more than I was ever taught. I found God/Goddess everywhere. I found God/Goddess in the bible, the Torah, The Tao, The Bhagavad Gita, and many other teachings. I found God/Goddess in teachings from other people. I found God/Goddess in nature. I found the answer to my question. The answer was yes. God/Goddess existed before and will exist long after we have left existence.

From there, I formed my belief system. It is simple. Life is for living. There is magic in every day we live. There is a God/Goddess. Jesus is a way cool dude! Holding on to that helped me get here. It got me past the mental abuse, the physical abuse, the chemical insanity, and the hell that is brought about by humanity.

I am a Christian. I am a believer in the creative force of existence.

Where can you find your own faith? Where can you find your own belief? I don't know. I don't have that answer.

I gave my son a poster for his Christmas present. It has a character from a video game, and it says, "Find Something To Believe In."

To me, that is the truth. Finding something to believe in gives you an anchor. It gives you moral direction. It keeps you honest. Most of all, it leads you on a path to truth. The religion is not important. It is your seeking God/Goddess that is important.

Even in my worst times. Even when I was broken and beaten and decimated mentally, Jesus was my dude. I had a compass and a direction. Cause Jesus was my dude!

It doesn't matter what path you take; find something to believe in. Live life! Because life is meant for living. It truly is beautiful. No matter where you are now. No matter what you have been through. You will see that you will find something to believe in one day.

I published most of my letters in this series anonymously. I hope they helped someone on their journey. I publish this one openly. There are three great powers in the world. They are Hope, Faith, and Love. I hope you find your path to faith and experience the love of life I have now.

Sincerely,

Elizabeth Walker

-Elizabeth Myers

The older I get, the more my definition of wellbeing tends to shift on all levels. I spent my childhood and teenage years with a complex set of survival skills and masking who I really was inside because my home was not a safe place to be me. Emotions were discouraged, and individuality was not welcomed. I learned survival instincts early, and my fight or flight was activated before I even left home.

I immediately searched for healing in all the wrong places. An older man who I married, and now that I look back, it was severe daddy issues and father wounds I needed to heal, but instead, I put a bandage on a significant problem. Because of that bandage, my wounds just seeped through, and new ones from an unhealed soul in a marriage just compounded the issues. After a roller-coaster ending to that marriage, I spent the next ten years trying to forget the marriage and the heartache inside me that I did not know how to fix. I wanted to find it at the bottom of the bottle, partying, broken men, and working myself into health issues for the pursuit of validation or accomplishment. Nothing worked. Once again, the problems only mounted one on the other until the weight was too much to carry anymore.

My fractured soul sought the approval of society and to fit in with a crowd that only rekindled the wounds I had deep within. Father wounds. Mother wounds. A lot of self-esteem issues and the pressure to still keep a mask on while being the person I was supposed to be. Normal, what even is normal by today's standards?

I was shamed for decisions I made while broken and coping unhealed with the trauma I had been left to fix on my own. Even though I started therapy within months of leaving my parent's home when I turned 18, it was still decades later, and while I could see progress, there was still a large part of me unhealed. I wanted to be better. I hated myself. I hated how I felt or the anger I could not control. I hated how much I felt things and how my emotions always got the best of me. I hated how kind-hearted I was and how people took advantage of it. I hated how I was left to raise children with no support from their father and that the support offered to me by others was stifled with conditions.

I went through abusive dating relationships and toxic friendships. All of which made me wonder if it was me; I was broken; I had to be the problem. Still, I could not see my way out. I tried to take my own life in desperation at one point – overwhelmed with the thought that everyone would be far better off if I was not around.

Years ticked by, and I tried to make better decisions. Working closer to home. I found work that allowed me a slightly better balance to provide for my kids, but I still see them some. Better work environments to lessen the stress. Spending time doing more things that brought me relaxation when I had a day off. Once again, I could fool others but never myself. I knew I still cried daily. I knew I still had anger and abandonment issues that I could not fix. I still was grieving for a life I was never meant to have. I kept a small circle of friends, and it seemed like whenever someone got too close, I either pushed them away or they betrayed me in a way that I deleted them from my life.

In my mid-thirties, I landed an excellent job close to home and made great money. It was a lot more scheduled than sporadic with hours. I had a balance in my home life and work life. As usual, I performed well at work. It was all about the validation I needed from my job, and I did almost anything I could to reach that (short of sleeping my way to the top). I mean, it was genuinely demanding and perfectionistic work. However, at this job, I found someone who wanted to date me, and I refused to do so because I was not going to risk my career, which I had carefully built to erode it over a man. He quit his job when I told him I wouldn't date him, and his love bombed me hard to make me believe his love was real. The crazy part I saw right from the start was that I NEVER loved him. I remember even as we started to date, I told my closest girlfriends that I didn't love him, but if he loved me so much, I would take it because I never wanted to love someone as deeply as I did before and lose them – I wasn't sure I could live through that again – and this gal, was playing it safe now.

Right off the start, I noticed red flags, but I excused them away. When I asked others, they excused it away for me. And so, I stayed. I lost my job. My world slowly crumbled piece by piece. I questioned my sanity. I worried for our lives. I was sick all the time. During one of the many sessions with my therapist while trying to create a safe plan to escape - she told me to imagine what my home would feel like if it was safe. How would it feel? What would it look like? Really visualize it. I did that so many times a day to keep my sanity.

Needless to say, that relationship and marriage ended up being the worst decision I had ever made in my entire life up to that point. It was seven years of indescribable abuse and losing myself in the process. Leaving that all behind, I created a new life for myself and my children – absent of the violence and abuse we had faced for those long years, but healing did not happen immediately. It had taken root in all of our lives, from nightmares to low self-esteem.

I had no way of remembering who I was before I met him. I knew I would never be her again. There were large chunks of time I could not even remember, and I didn't know if it was trauma or the cancer I had battled, robbing me of my mind. At that moment, I also realized that if there was ever a time I could totally revamp my life to look like what I really wanted it to look like, it would be now. I had a clean slate. I had lost everything. I could live where I chose to live. I could go by whatever name I liked most, explore all the hobbies I had put off doing in the past years, decorate my home how I loved it, and even wear a different style of clothes. I could be a new person and no longer had to be the person I was before.

It was a release almost to know I no longer had to keep up a mask or pretend to be someone I was not. I no longer needed validation or people to love me. I spent a lot of time healing myself, my trauma, my anger, my grief, my wounds, and my core being. My sole focus was on me. My healing. My safe space. My peace. A home where my children could also safely exist. It became a roadmap that I am still exploring as I write this. I have pushed myself to have better boundaries, to recognize toxic or abusive patterns, to release anxiety over what I cannot control, and to expand myself in directions I had never even thought of going. I remember realizing I had reached a moment I had not felt since I was a very young child. I was meditating while lying in bed – when the guided meditation said to bring yourself to the last time you remembered feeling the safest you have ever felt. I immediately thought, "That it is now!" That realization brought tears to my eyes. I felt safe. Actually, safe. Not surviving. Not masking. Not pretending. I felt SAFE. And that was worth it all.

Today, my life looks different. I dress in things that are comfy and that I love. It is up to me if I want my hair to be curly or straight. I have made my home a creative, safe space. I have explored alternative opportunities for living, school, and even my health. For the first time since 2016, I went to the doctor this month and was told my labs were perfect. Something I thought I might never hear again. I am off almost all medications because they are not needed. I go to a therapist. I have a circle of friends that align with my values.

My fibromyalgia never flares up. My migraines are less than ever. I sleep all night. I eat healthier. I walk everywhere. I relax. I do not stress. I let go of worry or anxiety. I am grateful. I don't feel I must keep my phone on or near me. I do not have to be active on social media unless I want to be. I do not have to answer someone immediately or do everything on my to-do list. I pace myself to what I can do. What I want to do. I enjoy the small moments in life. I allow for interruptions. If my children want to watch a movie at 10 in the morning, we do that. I use my energy for advocacy and giving back to the community. I do things every single day that I love to do. I spend time with my kids doing all the things they want to do. I work less. I live on less. I have learned that what I need to live is far less than most think. I am content. I slow down. And most of all – I take care of myself.

If I want an extra cup of coffee – I have it.

If I want to sleep in every day – I sleep in.

If I want to walk to the beach, I walk there.

If I want to dance – I dance.

72

If I want a hot bath – I take a hot bath.

No matter what – I live each day as if it were my last. In doing that, I have found that my wellbeing flows into all areas and is easily maintained.

I know you might read this and think – I cannot just start over with a clean slate, but I implore you – can you not? Or are you afraid of letting go of all that society pushes on us that is "important" and bringing yourself to the front of the line as a priority. Are you afraid of what might happen if you stopped in the rat race of life and actually LIVED? What might the silence bring up? What materialism you might discard? What false belief structures might collapse?

A wise woman once told me to ask myself, when stressed, "Is it an emergency? If it does not happen today, will someone die? Will someone not eat? Will your family not have shelter or safety? If the answer is no – then let it go for today." Wiser words have never been spoken because the moment I stripped my life down to the necessities and realized the bubble I had been in…I will never return to it. I love my simple life and knowing that I can have balance because I chose that road so that my wellbeing stays safely in place. Does it mean I do not have stress or worry or anxiety moments? Of course not. I still have them, but my reaction to them is different and in that, I do not let them control me or even have a front seat in my life anymore.

If you are unhappy and unfulfilled in your life – change it. Move. Start over. Do the things that scare you the most and in it you will find a happiness, contentment, and peace you never thought existed.

Choose you.

Choose your wellbeing.

It is the best decision you will ever make.

I promise.

-Blair Hayse

My Journey: Ellie Taylor Fani

It had been six months since I left my apartment...meaning I didn't leave my house for six months on end. Of course, one might think, why? Was there a specific reason? I remember where it all started. My brother was diagnosed with COVID a few weeks before it all started... there was something off in terms of how I was feeling. I decided to get tested to be on the safe side. Since there was a high demand for COVID tests and Urgent Care did not have rapid tests then, I took the PCR COVID test, which takes 24-48 hours to get your results back, sometimes less. I remember sleeping in my room, social distancing myself from my family just in case I had it. My mother and brother knocked on my door and came in. They didn't have the best expressions on their face. I remember when my mom told me I tested positive, and I just knew that was the start of a journey of emotions and recovery.

The first incident that happened after my COVID diagnosis was when I was fully recovered and hanging out with my mom. I was in my room, and at the time, I still had a very unhealthy attachment to my mom. I would either sleep in her room, or she would sleep in mine. I was in bed, and since it was during the COVID-19 breakout, I had hand sanitizer with me wherever I went. Hand sanitizer was sitting next to my water, and it was the type of hand sanitizer bottle that you had to push down to get some. In the span of two minutes, I convinced myself that hand sanitizer had gotten into my water. I was drinking the water, and since the mind has power, I didn't only think it fell in, but I also tasted it. A lot of the time when I tell this story, I myself find it silly, but it was such a real and powerful anxiety that it wasn't just a stupid thought I had. I went on, woke my mom up, and told her the situation. She took about 5-7 minutes to explain to me why that wasn't rational or possible. At the end of the conversation, I was still fixated on the possibility of me drinking hand sanitizer. I take it into my own hands and decide to look up what could happen if one ingested hand sanitizer and if I should go to the ER. I remember heading to bed hoping I would wake up the next morning, which again sounds silly, but it was so real and mind-boggling. I remember many other instances where I would convince myself of irrational things and scare myself during the process. I couldn't sit on my own furniture because I thought it was dirty; if my mom made me a meal, the plate could not touch the table or any surface I wasn't sure of; if something dirty touched the sheet, I would automatically ask to change it. Sometimes, I would change into pajamas and go to the bathroom, and my shirt would touch the sink, and I would have to change again. I couldn't turn the faucet on, I couldn't touch the bottles of shampoo and conditioner, I couldn't touch anything besides my phone, my mother's bed, and anything I thought was undoubtedly dirty. I washed my hands so often that my skin became irritated and red. There were ongoing arguments between my family and I. It was such a frustrating time. I didn't know what to do or how to get out of this unhealthy cycle. Sometimes, I didn't know if I wanted to fight anymore. I didn't want to keep going like this.

I had been diagnosed with OCD (Obsessive Compulsive Disorder) and anxiety after my first COVID diagnosis. I went to therapy and eventually got on medication. I remember going over everything I had ever been anxious about regarding germs. She was by far the best therapist I had ever had and talked to. She gave me coping mechanisms to use when I would start freaking out, and she gave me tasks to achieve every week that had to do with germs. Whether that be refraining from cleaning my phone or getting myself to go outside. We would talk about how I want to get better and how I will achieve that. I got a psychiatrist, and we talked about different medications that help with OCD. I was prescribed Fluoxetine, which had excellent results when it came to those with OCD and depression. I didn't want medicine to be my last resort, but I can say now that it was definitely a lifesaver, and I am more than grateful to have gone on it. I found myself getting outside more, freaking out less, touching things without having to wash my hands, and part of the reason I got outside after six months was because of the help that my family, friends, and therapist gave me.

I remember vividly when my brother's former girlfriend was determined to help me escape the fear and overwhelming feeling of this. For the first time in six months, I went outside and sat on our building steps with shorts on. This was a huge step for me because, at the time, I convinced myself that if I sat anywhere but my mother's bed, I would get sick and die.

My parents tried their best to understand what was going on with me psychologically. My mom is a therapist, making it easier to understand where I was coming from. She did her best even in the most difficult times. Sometimes, she would try to use exposure therapy with me. She tried to help me research OCD to understand it better. And sometimes, she would get upset and lose her patience. It was so understandable as to why she lost her patience. It was an everyday thing, and it was an all-day thing. I mean, I did wake her up at night more often than I'd like to admit. My dad was both supportive of me and frustrated because he didn't really understand the nuances of OCD. I often had to sit down and explain to my parents what went through my head, even if it made no sense. There were times when I said, "I know you don't understand it, but this is what goes through my head, and I need you to respect that. I need you to try and understand it and I need you to prevent triggering me. They both did their best with what they knew at the time. My brother was the only one who ever really kept his patience. He listened to my concerns and answered my questions to the best of his ability. It wasn't only my family and doctors but also friends. One of my best friends from Connecticut came to New York City to visit me. She knew I couldn't touch certain things, but at this time, I could go outside. She was the most understanding out of anyone. She would ask me if she could touch me, if she could sit in places, and what she should do to make me comfortable, and she would reassure me when I was in the midst of a panic attack. I remember her being the first person I hugged after those harsh six months. I felt so safe.

With the help of therapy, the support of my friends and family, medication, and prayer, I got better. I could finally go out in the spring of that long, crucial year. And now, I go everywhere you could imagine, and I touch things that, three years ago, I would swear not to touch. I go to Westchester, I sit in cars, I sit on public transportation, I sit on the concrete in New York City (ew.), I sit on my furniture, and now I am the most independent individual I can be. I have started traveling by myself, which feels fantastic. I have a job now and help hundreds of people daily. It feels good.

Sometimes, I'll come across a photo of me and my mom at the Natural History Museum park, and I just look at it and smile. It means a lot to know I got through one of the most challenging times of my life, even when I didn't think I would make it out. I'm grateful for how far I've come, and I wanted to offer you, the person reading this, the hope that things can get better and time heals. I didn't know how I would be able to live my life, but something shifted. I worked hard on my healing and growth.

I am writing this letter to show others my experience and prove it has improved. Please believe in yourself, try your best, communicate, ask for help, and do not give up. You will make it through. I'm here to see if I can support you in any way. If you need advice or support, please email me at elisabettataylorfani@gmail.com.

Thank you for reading this,
Ellie

-Ellie Taylor Fani

APPENDIX ON SUPPORT RESOURCES & CHOICES

Includes Tips & Resources For Emotional, Physical, & Spiritual Wellbeing

Tips for Enhancing your Emotional, Physical, & Spiritual Wellbeing
Originally published in Girl on Fire Magazine by Jen Taylor, LCSW

Manifesting involves living the life we want as though we already have it.

Act the part.
Be confident.
You've got this ALREADY!
Don't say "I am trying." Or "I am working on this." Use " I AM" statements like "I am a happy human."

Invest time, money, and energy in yourself every day.
Invest in that therapy session, that manicure, that networking lunch.
You are worth it.

Use positive thoughts to change your feelings.
Instead of doubting and saying "I don't know how I'll ever get there," change your mindset, say instead "These are bumps on the road to my success story!"

Don't forget to hydrate!
Get enough sleep!
Meditate - even five minutes a day helps!
Love yourself!!
You are your best investment!!!

Be Kind - To Yourself

So much of present-day society focuses on the external: our social media pages, what we look like, what we own, and where we work. However, the true measure of success lies in how we feel about ourselves internally.

Cognitive behavioral therapy suggests that our thoughts determine our feelings.

How do you talk to yourself on a daily basis?

Are you self-critical?

Are you internalizing someone else's judgmental voice?

If you are, don't give up hope. We all have voices from the past (a parent or teacher or sibling) that are not the kindest. It takes time to turn these negative messages around. Take a few minutes today to listen to your self-talk. If you find that it is negative or judgmental, try talking back.

For example, if the negative self-talk is saying, "I am a bad mom," take a moment to respond. You might say, "I am not a bad mom. I am doing my best. I am a loving, dedicated mom who sometimes has a hard day." Doing this takes practice. However, with time, you will find that it becomes easier and more natural.

Isn't it ironic how easily we can find the right, supportive words with our kids or friends when they are struggling? We are most definitely the hardest on ourselves. We would never dream of judging a dear one the way we judge ourselves.

Work on becoming your own "top fan." When you've done a fantastic job, tell yourself how awesome you are and how proud you are. You might say, "Wow. That was a tough situation, and I handled it beautifully." Or, "Let's reward ourselves with something for getting through that horrendous day!" One exercise for you to practice is to stand in front of the mirror and say three positive affirmations. These can be anything from "I have beautiful eyes" to "I am a committed and understanding friend." Initially, this can feel very vulnerable, but with time and practice, it will get easier and give a boost to your day. If you are uncomfortable standing in front of a mirror, try writing in a "gratitude journal." Give thanks every day for three things in your life. Focusing on the positive has a way of making magic happen. It is clinically proven that changing our thoughts can improve our feelings.

Our belief in ourselves is the root of our success in all aspects of life. It is a relationship we must cultivate. Sometimes, when feeling blue, try to connect with your inner child and ask what he/she/they need.

A little more rest?

A brownie?

Or a cuddle?

Even as an adult try to maintain a self-care routine…that can be anything such as: salt baths, daily time to yourself, and weekly lessons with a spiritual teacher. This can be hard when we have younger or special needs children. Even 30 minutes alone will do wonders if you can swing it.

One last self-care reminder is to be kind and gentle with ourselves. God knows it's a challenging world out there. We need to be in our own corner.

NAMI Helpline (National Alliance on Mental Illness) 1-800-950-6264

APPENDIX ON SUICIDE RESOURCES

Includes Resources for

Suicide Help & Assessment

List of Suicide Help & Hotlines[1]:
(United States and Worldwide)

United States:
Emergency: 911
Suicide Hotline: 988

Algeria:
Emergency: 34342 and 43
Suicide Hotline: 0021 3983 2000 58

Angola:
Emergency: 113

Argentina:
Emergency: 911
Suicide Hotline: 135

Armenia:
Emergency: 911 and 112
Suicide Hotline: (2) 538194

---

[1] List of Helplines and Hotline Numbers Retrieved from blog.opencounseling.com

Australia:
Emergency: 000
Suicide Hotline: 131114

Austria:
Emergency: 112
Telefonseelsorge 24/7 142
Rat auf Draht 24/7 147 (Youth)

Bahamas:
Emergency: 911
Suicide Hotline: (2) 322-2763

Bahrain:
Emergency: 999

Bangladesh:
Emergency: 999

Barbados:
Emergency: 911
Suicide Hotline Samaritan Barbados: (246) 4299999

Belgium:
Emergency: 112
Suicide Hotline Stichting Zelfmoordlijn: 1813

Bolivia:
Emergency: 911
Suicide Hotline: 3911270

Bosnia & Herzegovina:
Suicide Hotline: 080 05 03 05

Botswana:
Emergency: 911
Suicide Hotline: +2673911270

Brazil:
Emergency: 188

Bulgaria:
Emergency: 112
Suicide Hotline: 0035 9249 17 223

Burundi:
Emergency: 117

Burkina Faso:
Emergency: 17

Canada:
Emergency: 911
Suicide Hotline: 1 (822) 456 4566

Chad:
Emergency: 2251-1237

China:
Emergency: 110
Suicide Hotline: 800-810-1117

Columbia:
24/7 Helpline in Barranquilla: 1(00 57 5) 372 27 27
24/7 Hotline Bogota: (57-1 323 24 25

Congo:
Emergency: 117

Costa Rica:
Emergency: 911
Suicide Hotline: 506-253-5439

Croatia:
Emergency: 112

Cyprus:
Emergency: 112
Suicide Hotline: 8000 7773

Czech Republic:
Emergency: 112

Denmark:
Emergency: 112
Suicide Hotline: 4570201201

Dominican Republic:
Emergency: 911
Suicide Hotline: (809) 562-3500

Ecuador:
Emergency: 911

Egypt:
Emergency: 122
Suicide Hotline: 131114

El Salvador:
Emergency: 911
Suicide Hotline: 126

Equatorial Guinea:
Emergency: 114

Estonia:
Emergency:112
Suicide Hotline: 3726558088
In Russian: 3726555688

Ethiopia:
Emergency: 911

Finland:
Emergency: 112
Suicide Hotline: 010 195 202

France:
Emergency: 112
Suicide Hotline: 0145394000

Germany:
Emergency: 112
Suicide Hotline: 0800 111 0 111

Ghana:
Emergency: 999
Suicide Hotline: 2332 444 71279

Greece:
Emergency: 1018

Guatemala:
Emergency: 110
Suicide Hotline: 5392-5953

Guinea:
Emergency: 117

Guinea Bissau:
Emergency: 117

Guyana:
Emergency: 999
Suicide Hotline: 223-0001

Holland:
Suicide Hotline: 09000767

Hong Kong:
Emergency: 999
Suicide Hotline: 852 2382 0000

Hungary:
Emergency: 112
Suicide Hotline: 116123

India:
Emergency: 112
Suicide Hotline: 8888817666

Indonesia:
Emergency: 112
Suicide Hotline: 1-800-273-8255

Iran:
Emergency: 110
Suicide Hotline: 1480

Ireland:
Emergency: 116123
Suicide Hotline: +4408457909090

Israel:
Emergency: 100
Suicide Hotline: 1201

Italy:
Emergency: 112
Suicide Hotline: 800860022

Jamaica:
Suicide Hotline: 1-888-429-KARE (5273)

Japan:
Emergency: 110
Suicide Hotline: 810352869090

Jordan:
Emergency: 911
Suicide Hotline: 110

Kenya:
Emergency: 999
Suicide Hotline: 722178177

Kuwait:
Emergency: 112
Suicide Hotline: 94069304

Latvia:
Emergency: 113
Suicide Hotline: 371 67222922

Lebanon:
Suicide Hotline: 1564

Liberia:
Emergency: 911
Suicide Hotline: 6534308

Luxembourg:
Emergency: 112
Suicide Hotline: 352 45 45 45

Madagascar:
Emergency: 117

Malaysia:
Emergency: 999
Suicide Hotline: (06) 2842500

Mali:
Emergency: 8000-1115

Malta:
Suicide Hotline: 179

Mauritius:
Emergency: 112
Suicide Hotline: +230 800 93 93

Mexico:
Emergency: 911
Suicide Hotline: 5255102550

Netherlands:
Emergency: 112

Suicide Hotline: 900 0113

New Zealand:
Emergency: 111
Suicide Hotline: 1737

Niger:
Emergency: 112

Nigeria:
Suicide Hotline: 234 8092106493

Norway:
Emergency: 112
Suicide Hotline: +4781533300

Pakistan:
Emergency: 115

Peru:
Emergency: 911
Suicide Hotline: 381-3695

Philippines:
Emergency: 911
Suicide Hotline: 028969191

Poland:
Emergency: 112
Suicide Hotline: 5270000

Portugal:
Emergency: 112
Suicide Hotline: 21 854 07 40

And 8 96 898 21 50

Qatar:
Emergency: 999

Romania:
Emergency: 112
Suicide Hotline: 0800 801200

Russia:
Emergency: 112
Suicide Hotline: 0078202577577

Saint Vincent and the Grenadines:
Suicide Hotline: 9784 456 1044

São Tomé and Príncipe:
Suicide Hotline: (239) 222-12-22 ext. 123

Saudi Arabia:
Emergency: 112

Serbia:
Suicide Hotline: (+381) 21-6623-393

Senegal:
Emergency: 17

Singapore:
Emergency: 999
Suicide Hotline: 1 800 2214444

Spain:
Emergency: 112

Suicide Hotline: 914590050

South Africa:
Emergency: 10111
Suicide Hotline: 0514445691

South Korea:
Emergency: 112
Suicide Hotline: (02) 7158600

Sri Lanka:
Suicide Hotline: 011 057 2222662

Sudan:
Suicide Hotline: (249) 11-555-253

Sweden:
Emergency: 112
Suicide Hotline: 46317112400

Switzerland:
Emergency: 112
Suicide Hotline: 143

Tanzania:
Emergency: 112

Thailand:
Suicide Hotline: (02) 713-6793

Tonga:
Suicide Hotline: 23000

Trinidad and Tobago:
Suicide Hotline: (868) 645 2800

Tunisia:
Emergency: 197

Turkey:
Emergency: 112

Uganda:
Emergency: 112
Suicide Hotline: 0800 21 21 21

United Arab Emirates:
Suicide Hotline: 800 46342

United Kingdom:
Emergency: 112
Suicide Hotline: 0800 689 5652

United States:
Emergency: 911
Suicide Hotline: 988

Zambia:
Emergency: 999
Suicide Hotline: +260960264040

Zimbabwe:
Emergency: 999
Suicide Hotline: 080 12 333 333

CONDUCT A SUICIDE INQUIRY[2]

a. Ideation

Frequency, Intensity and Duration

- Have you had thoughts of hurting yourself or others?
- Have you thought about ending your life?

Now, in the Past, and at its Worst

- During the last 48 hours, past month, and worst ever: How much? How intense? Lasting for how long?

b. Plan

Timing, Location, Lethality, Availability/Means

- When you think about killing yourself or ending your life, what do you imagine?
- When? Where? How would you do it? In what way?

Preparatory Acts

- What steps have you taken to prepare to kill yourself, if any?

---

[2] Retrieved from Minnesota Department of Health at: https://www.health.state.mn.us/people/syringe/suicide.pdf

c. Behavior

Past attempts, aborted attempts, rehearsals

- Have you ever thought about or tried to kill yourself in the past?
- Have you ever taken any actions to rehearse or practice ending your life (e.g., tying noose, loading gun, measuring substance)?

Non-suicidal self-injurious behavior

- Are you having paranoid thoughts? Hallucinations?
- Have you done anything to hurt yourself (e.g., cutting, burning or mutilation)?

d. Intent

Extent to which they expect to carry out the plan and believe the plan to be lethal versus harmful.

- What do you think will happen?
- What things put you at risk of ending your life or killing yourself (reasons to die)?
- What things prevent you from killing yourself and keep you safe (reasons to live)?

Explore ambivalence between reasons to die and reasons to live. Pay attention to how they describe the outcome.

- "I'm dead, it's over." indicates a higher risk of suicide death.

- "I think I'd end up in the hospital." indicates a moderate risk of suicide death.
- "I don't want to die; I want my suffering to end." indicates a lower risk of suicide death.

e. Notes

- When working with **youth**, collect information from a parent, guardian or service provider on the youth's suicidal thoughts, plans, behaviors, and changes in mood, behavior or disposition.
- If the person has thoughts or plans to **harm someone else**, conduct a homicide inquiry using the same questions (replace "hurt or kill yourself" with "hurt or kill someone else").

DETERMINE RISK LEVEL[3]

The risk level is determined with the previous three steps:

1. Risk Factors
2. Protective Factors
3. Suicide Inquiry

Death by Suicide Risk Level

Risk Level	Risk Factors	Protective Factors	Suicide Inquiry	Intervention*
High	Multiple risk factors	Protective factors are not present or not relevant at this time	Potentially lethal suicide attempt or persistent ideation with strong intent or suicide rehearsal	Hospital admission generally indicated, suicide precautions (e.g., observation, means reduction)
Moderate	Multiple risk factors	Few protective factors	Suicidal ideation with a plan, but not intent or behavior	Hospital admission may be necessary, develop crisis plan and suicide precautions, give emergency/crisis numbers

---

[3] Retrieved from Minnesota Department of Health at:
https://www.health.state.mn.us/people/syringe/suicide.pdf

	Few and/or modifiable risk factors	Strong protective factors	Thoughts of death with no plan, intent or behavior	Outpatient referral, symptom reduction, give emergency/crisis numbers
Low				

Take every suicide attempt seriously!

People often think a person is not really suicidal.

It's better to be safe, even if they will be angry with you for taking action to keep them alive.

ABOUT THE AUTHOR

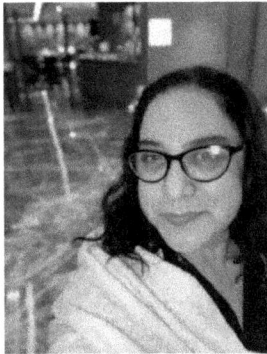

Jen Taylor, LCSW
#1 International Bestselling Author

Jen Taylor, LCSW is a New York-based spiritual psychotherapist with 23+ years of experience. Jen specializes in womens' empowerment, domestic violence, teens, and LGBTQIA+ individuals. Jen incorporates spirituality and astrology into her sessions to create a truly unique blend of guidance.

Jen was born and raised in New York City and lived there from preschool through high school. Instead of attending her prom, Jen went to boot camp for the Navy and received accreditation as a U.S. Naval photographer. Jen then received her Bachelor's in Arts from Haverford College in Pennsylvania and studied abroad in Florence, Italy. She spent her early 20s in the advertising office of Italian *Vogue* and went on to attend social work school at Fordham University's Graduate school of social services. In 1999, Jen received her Master's in social work while pregnant with her first child, Giancarlo. Jen worked in various outpatient mental health clinics in New York City, and in 2007 had her second child, Elisabetta.

Jen Taylor, LCSW is the editor for Girl on Fire Magazine's "Wine Down with Jen," where she uses her 20+ years of experience as a New York-based spiritual psychotherapist to bring you cozy couch conversations you would have with your best friend over a glass of wine after work.

When not writing for the magazine or seeing clients, Jen enjoys traveling, photography, spending time with her kids, and a good cup of coffee.

Jen is a multiple #1 International bestselling author in a collaboration series and currently working on releasing the rest of this series as her very first solo books over the next year.

To connect with Jen, she can be reached at:

Jentaylorfani@gmail.com

www.ingramcontent.com/pod-product-compliance
Lightning Source LLC
Chambersburg PA
CBHW071240020426
42333CB00015B/1556